Student Recruitment in Psychosocial Occupational Therapy: Intergenerational Approaches

T0186832

Student Recruitment in Psychosocial Occupational Therapy: Intergenerational Approaches

Susan Haiman
Editor

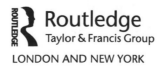

Routledge
Taylor & Francis Group

LONDON AND NEW YORK

First published 1990 by Haworth Press, Inc.

Published 2018 by Routledge
2 Park Square, Milton Park, Abingdon, Oxon OX14 4RN
52 Vanderbilt Avenue, New York, NY 10017

First issued in paperback 2018

Routledge is an imprint of the Taylor & Francis Group, an informa business

Student Recruitment in Psychosocial Occupational Therapy: Intergenerational Approaches has also been published as *Occupational Therapy in Mental Health*, Volume 10, Number 1 1990.

Library of Congress Cataloging-in-Publication Data

Student recruitment in psychosocial occupational therapy : intergenerational approaches / Susan Haiman, guest editor.
    p. cm.
Has also been published as Occupational therapy in mental health, v. 10, no. 1, 1990.
Includes bibliographical references.
ISBN 0-86656-993-6
    1. Occupational therapists — Recruiting. 2. Occupational therapy — Study and teaching.
RM735.4.S78   1990
615.8′515′0711 – dc20   90-4541
                                                     CIP

ISBN 13: 978-1-138-87318-6 (pbk)
ISBN 13: 978-0-86656-993-4 (hbk)

Student Recruitment in Psychosocial Occupational Therapy: Intergenerational Approaches

CONTENTS

ABOUT THE EDITOR

Susan Haiman, MPS, OTR/L, is Assistant Director of Therapeutic Activities at Payne Whitney Clinic, New York Hospital, and Lecturer in Psychiatry at Cornell Medical Center, New York City. She has been a clinical educator, supervisor, and administrator in mental health settings since 1971. Her expertise in clinical reasoning and decision making in the areas of individual and group treatment planning and intervention has been critical to the roles she has assumed as clinician, program developer, and manager. She has lectured and published papers in these areas as well.

Ms. Haiman is a registered occupational therapist and holds a Master's in Public Services in Health Services Administration and Mental Health Management. She is a member of the American Occupational Therapy Association and has served as faculty on the "Focus on Mental Health: Skills for Assessment and Treatment." She is also a member of the New York State Occupational Therapy Association. Ms. Haiman serves on the editorial board of *Occupational Therapy in Mental Health* and is a reviewer for *Hospital and Community Psychiatry*.

Preface

Education and Enticement:
A Recruitment Strategy

Susan Haiman, MPS, OTR/L

The Mental Health Special Interest Section of The American Occupational Therapy Association (AOTA) has identified recruitment and retention of occupational therapists into mental health as a critical concern in the coming year (Dickie, 1989). It is no surprise to those practicing in the psychosocial arena that it has become increasingly difficult to meet service demands due to the shortage of occupational therapists to fill available positions. In fact, the entire profession faces similar difficulties as the college age population decreases and the pool of potential students diminishes, leaving fewer and fewer resources at the entry level (Johnson, 1981; Masatagani, 1986). The impact of this was cited by Bonder (1987) who wrote of a dramatic decline in the numbers of occupational therapists employed in community mental health centers. Indicating that occupational therapy in mental health has not kept pace with other areas of specialty practice.

The time has come to devote our energy toward recognizing factors that lead individuals to select occupational therapy as a profession, and mental health as an area of specialization. Practicing therapists and educators must focus on these influencing factors and build upon them to encourage, promote, and support those individuals with identified competence and growing interest in particular

Susan Haiman is Assistant Director, Department of Therapeutic Activities, and Lecturer, Department of Psychiatry, Payne Whitney Clinic-Cornell Medical Center, 525 East 68th Street, New York, NY 10021.

ix

areas. The task of insuring competence and adequate manpower can not simply be left to our leadership. All of us must help to devise creative solutions that will "activate new levels of capability to meet the demands of the public" (Serrett, 1985, p.3). We must begin to target specific populations for recruitment, such as those cited by the AOTA Ad Hoc Commission on Occupational Therapy Manpower, e.g., second career students, underemployed students from other related fields, minority students, special needs students and men (Masatagani, 1986, p.525).

Not only must we think about at whom recruitment strategies must be directed; consideration must be given to reviewing what we offer new recruits to entice them into the profession and into psychosocial practice: a sound education; a process of professional socialization and an opportunity to develop a professional identity; role models; mentoring relationships; and the richest Level I and Level II fieldwork experiences available. The following pages will focus briefly on each of these "offerings" by way of introduction to the main body of content in this special issue.

Johnson (1981), wrote that the recruitment of people was not sufficient to insuring increased manpower. Keeping pace with the definition of conceptual problems and developing sound theoretical frameworks is also critical to the ability to attract and keep students in the profession. The mandate is that we value the knowledge base we have, share it and use it for support, nurturance and to open doors for ourselves and our students (Johnson, 1981).

Fidler (1979), writing about the educational implications of specialization, called upon educators to constantly review, critique and explore ways in which students develop "intellectual, manual and interpersonal skills" (p.35) relevant to the selected specialty and the "concomitant art of application" (p.35). Fidler, in the same article stated that educators must provide experiences that "reinforce professional values, attitudes, critical thinking and autonomy" (p.35).

Some might be concerned that specialty selection early in the educational process will lead to fragmentation of the profession and its view of man. Slaymaker (1986), reminds us that despite pursuit of special interests, we can remain a holistic profession, where competence in any specialty area requires proficiency in psychosocial practice. Conversely, competence in psychosocial practice requires training and experience with "neurosensory function" (Slaymaker, 1986, p.120), as well as knowledge of the impact of physical, motor and developmental factors on function and treatment.

Finally, there is concern that psychosocial courses are not well taught and that students prefer concrete material to abstract, analytic material (Christie et al., 1985). There is also belief that practice in psychosocial arenas requires a greater level of maturity, as it is difficult to work in the affective domains (Christie et al., 1985, p.673). It falls on the shoulders of educators to be the first to dispel these misconceptions and reconcile the idealized images of the profession, as taught in the classroom, with the realities encountered in clinical settings (Sabari, 1985).

Clinicians, too have responsibility for linking classroom to clinic throughout the educational experience. As, in addition to acquiring professional knowledge, students also experience a process of professional socialization and identity building. Sabari (1985) identified those people who serve as socializing agents encountered by students during formal training: full time faculty; clinicians functioning as part-time instructors; physicians teaching background courses; and fieldwork supervisors (p.98). Furthermore, says Sabari, "Socializing influences to which students are exposed during their professional education may have greater impact on their future practice than the academic and clinical information they learn" (p.96). To insure effective socialization, fieldwork supervisors, academics and even upperclassmen within occupational therapy programs must find ways to help newcomers "develop healthy and consistent role adaptability, a hallmark of our profession," (Sabari, 1985, p.101-102).

The results of a study of Townsend and Mitchell (1982) indicated that personal contact was the most effective means of creating interest in occupational therapy. Extrapolating from these results, it is possible that increasing personal contact with occupational therapists in mental health will be an effective means of creating interest in this specialty area. Thus, in addition to socialization, every effort must be made to provide effective role models who, through professional behavior, can influence and encourage students to pursue mental health practice. Cavanaugh (1975) stated that role modelling after "mature teachers" has a powerful influence on trainee behavior and professional identity (p.277).

In 1986, Rogers described role modelling as an essentially passive mode of influence on career development. Students select role models from among those viewed as having skills and abilities students "lack, admire and want to emulate" (p.79). They then observe, imitate, identify with and evaluate their own learning in comparison to selected role models. Senior therapists, therefore, must be aware of the potential of becoming role models to students and younger therapists without having direct interaction with them. Fidler (1981) warned that, as theory continues to develop as crucial to the practice of occupational therapy, educators and practitioners should not forget that understanding the meaning of activity is critical to our sense of competence, and is the base of the profession which it is necessary to pass on, despite the fact that "in our western society, occupations employing verbal-cognitive skills are assigned greater value than those whose work involves manual skills" (p.570).

Finally, the potential for discovering a mentor must be available to recruits. Many believe that a mentor is essential to success in any field, and particularly in psychiatry where the demands of attempting to help "people who have a meaningless existence: people who are unable to use their time in purposeful activity" (Gillette, Kielhofner, 1979, p.22), can lead to feelings of "defeat, helplessness and loss of direction among trainees in any discipline faced continually with the need to recreate the wheel" (Dixon, 1989).

Mentoring was described by Rogers (1986) as a unique relationship in which the mentor takes a personal interest in a student: guiding, advising and nurturing him or her in very concrete ways. The mentor not only role models, but actively provides essential career information and opens doors of opportunity wherever possible (p.79). Students do not become clinical specialists through didactic teaching. Integration of theory and practice is "best cultivated by a close, prolonged one-to-one relationship" (Rogers, 1986, p.81). Occupational therapists in mental health have a unique opportunity to become mentors to those facing career decisions. This is an opportunity not to be taken lightly, as mentoring carries with it a strong personal commitment to accepting responsibility for helping a less experienced person develop; to sharing political know-how; and to communicating expertise in an exclusive fashion (Rogers, 1986).

Thus, mentorship relationships, in their truest sense, are not common, as one cannot easily function as a mentor to many. However, fieldwork experiences offer chance to develop such relationships within the context of supervision. An effective supervisory relationship contains all the essential components to turn a supervisor into mentor and a supervisee into "mentoree!" Heightened awareness of the powerful potential of this relationship carries an important message to all occupational therapists in mental health. The message is that each clinician is obligated to provide the best, most effective supervision possible, and, when desirable, to use that supervisory relationship as a recruitment strategy! Christie, Joyce and Moeller (1985) reported that greater than one half of the students they studied either selected or confirmed their specialty based on fieldwork experience. Ezersky, Havazelet, Scott and Zettler (1989), also reported a survey in which the quality of the fieldwork experience ranked first among reasons influencing specialty choice. What better evidence is needed to emphasize the importance of fieldwork supervision? What data presents a stronger case for providing students in Level II mental health fieldwork placements with enhanced opportunity for professional identity building, socialization, exposure to potential role models and to those who can offer mentoring relationships?

Therefore, it gives me great pleasure to introduce this special collection entitled, "Student Recruitment in Psychosocial Occupational Therapy: Intergenerational Approaches." This entire volume presents the background, methodology and content of a day long seminar for Level II fieldwork students at New York Hospital-Cornell Medical Center, Payne Whitney Clinic in New York, New York. The program, sponsored by the Department of Therapeutic Activities, coordinated by Winnie Ebb, MS, OTR/L and this author, was intended to introduce students to a wide range of career options in occupational therapy in mental health and to expose them to new role models, potential mentors and a day of professional socialization.

Special thanks goes to all twelve senior clinicians in mental health practice who willingly donated their time and expertise to making the day an apparent success. Though it is not possible to publish everyone's efforts, the following registered occupational therapists gave brief presentations on their special areas of expertise and interest: Arlene Michaelson Baily, MS, OTR/L, CRC, (prevocational services); Dawn Beverley, OTR/L and Ellen Rabinowitz, MPS, OTR/L, (occupational therapy with geriatric and Alzheimer's patients); Tina Barth, MA, OTR/L, CRC, (interventions with addictive personalities); Winnie Ebb, MS, OTR/L, (Model of Human Occupation in clinical practice and research); Nadine Revheim, MS, OTR/L, (occupational therapist as clinician, educator and student); Perri Stern, MA, OTR/L, (psychoeducation and alternative employment for occupational therapists); Joan Feder, MA, OTR/L, (role of professional associations); and this author, (treatment of hospitalized adolescents).

Readers of the following pages will find the lead article by Anne Hiller Scott, MA, OTR, FAOTA, who has written extensively on issues around specialty selection in occupational therapy. Her article entitled "A Review, Reflections and Recommendations: Specialty Preference of Mental Health in Occupational Therapy" provides a framework for the articles which follow. Next is an article titled "Enriching the Fieldwork II Experience: A Recruitment Strategy for Psychosocial Occupational Therapy," by Winnie Ebb, MS, OTR/L and this author, describing the rationale, methodology and outcome of the student seminar.

The final three articles are written versions of presentations contributed by individuals from three generations of mentors, role models and teachers. Each author has generously given time, energy, spirit and knowledge when serving as mentor for a few, role model for many, and knowledgeable leadership to the entire profession. Their contributions to the student seminar and to this volume are evidence of their willingness to share personal and professional philosophies regarding the vicissitudes of their own career paths in mental health specialty practice. Mark Rosenfeld, PhD, OTR/L, described his growth experiences and professional development in his article titled "A Mid-Career Perspective of Mental Health Practice." Through his writing one learns of moving from clinician to academic while sustaining a commitment to service, theory development and student education.

Susan B. Fine, MA, OTR, FAOTA, shares her thirty years of experience as practitioner, role model and mentor and how her professional growth was affected by the major trends in health care and specifically in mental health. Her paper titled "The Promise of Occupational Therapy: Professional Challenges, Personal Rewards" represents continued commitment to future generations of mental health specialists.

The final article was contributed by Gail Fidler, OTR/L, FAOTA, whose "Reflections on Choice" shares the wisdom and perspective of maturity with all readers. Her words address issues far beyond those related to specialty selection for occupational therapists, to present a philosophy which can guide anyone believing in and aspiring to independent, autonomous decision making in their personal and professional lives.

Before readers turn to the main body of this journal, take a moment to look backward. These words, spoken by Dr. Adolph Meyer, testified that a founder of our profession, Eleanore Clarke Slagle, was one of its finest teachers, role models, mentors, and a most effective recruiter! In 1937, Dr. Meyer said:

> It is a great privilege to speak on this occasion which honors . . . Mrs. Eleanore Clarke Slagle, as a person and as the personification of occupational therapy . . . she has been . . . a leader by example . . .
>
> Obviously, Mrs. Slagle has had her ideal not only in perpetuating herself in a special role but in training a rank and file ever able to furnish timber for leadership from the ranks and in the ranks, and growth from the ranks (p.109). . . .

REFERENCES

Bonder, B. (1987). Occupational therapy in mental health: Crisis or opportunity. American Journal of Occupational Therapy. 41(8), 495-499.

Cavanaugh, J.D. (1975). Career decisions in the early postresidency year. American Journal of Psychiatry. 132(3), 277-280.

Christie, B.A., Joyce, P.C., & Moeller, P.L. (1985). Fieldwork experience part

I: Impact on practice preference. American Journal of Occupational Therapy. 39(10), 671-674.

Dickie, V. (1989). Mental Health Special Interest Section Proceedings. Baltimore, MD: American Occupational Therapy Association National Conference.

Dixon, L. (1989). Personal Communication. New York, N.Y.

Dunn, W., Rask, S. (1989). Entry level and specialized practice. American Journal of Occupational Therapy. 43(1), 7-10.

Ezersky, S., Havazelet, L., Scott, A.H., & Zettler, C.L.B. (1989). Specialty choice in occupational therapy. American Journal of Occupational Therapy. 43(4), 227-233.

Fidler, G. (1979). Specialization: Implications for education. American Journal of Occupational Therapy. 33(1), 34-35.

Fidler, G.S. (1981). From crafts to competence. American Journal of Occupational Therapy. 35(9), 567-573.

Frum, D.C., Opacich, K.J. (1987). Supervision: Development of therapeutic competence. Rockville, MD: Rush University and the American Occupational Therapy Association.

Gillette, N., Kielhofner, G. (1979). The impact of specialization on the professionalization and survival of occupational therapy. American Journal of Occupational Therapy. 33(1), 20-28.

Johnson, N. (1981). Old values — new directions: Competence, adaptation, integration. American Journal of Occupational Therapy. 35(9), 589-598.

Masagatani, G. (1986). AOTA'S ad hoc commission on occupational therapy manpower. American Journal of Occupational Therapy. 40(8), 525-527.

Meyer, A. (1985). Address in honor of Eleanore Clarke Slagle. Occupational Therapy in Mental Health. 5(3), 109-113.

Montgomery, M.A., Evert, M.M., Kawar, M.J. (1979). In this issue. American Journal of Occupational Therapy. 33(1), 14.

Rogers, J.C. (1986). Mentoring for career achievement and advancement. American Journal of Occupational Therapy. 40(3), 79-82.

Sabari, J.S. (1985). Professional socialization: Implications for occupational therapy. American Journal of Occupational Therapy. 39(2), 96-102.

Scott, A.H. (1989). A Review, reflections and recommendations: Specialty, preference of mental health in occupational therapy. Occupational Therapy in Mental Health. This issue.

Serrett, K.D. (1985). Another look at occupational therapy's history: Paradigm or pair-of-hands. Occupational Therapy in Mental Health. 5(3), 1-32.

Shalik, H., Shalik, L. (1988). The occupational therapy level II fieldwork experience: Estimation of the fiscal benefit. American Journal of Occupational Therapy. 45(3), 164-168.

Slaymaker, J.H. (1986). A holistic approach to specialization. American Journal of Occupational Therapy. 40(2), 117-121.

Townsend, K.R., Mitchell, M.M. (1982). Effectiveness of recruitment and information techniques in occupational therapy. American Journal of Occupational Therapy. 36(8), 524-529.

A Review, Reflections
and Recommendations:
Specialty Preference of Mental Health
in Occupational Therapy

Anne Hiller Scott, MA, OTR, FAOTA

SUMMARY. It is sobering to consider that the majority of occupational therapy students have fieldwork experiences in mental health and physical disabilities and yet less than 15% choose practice in mental health. How can one account for the limited interest of students in mental health in a field that strongly espouses a holistic approach to patients? This article explores and reviews potential parameters affecting the specialty choice of mental health, to encourage further clarification of problems, identify areas for research and foster creative problem solving. Several theoretical lenses will be suggested to promote clearer focus on conceptual approaches to understanding practice preferences. The occupational therapy literature will be reviewed focusing on personality characteristics, learning style, academic and fieldwork experience and job satisfaction. Additional perspectives including specialization, reality shock, and discontinuity between the academic and clinical phases of professional training are offered from the literature on professional socialization as viable models for understanding this phenomenon. To reverse the trend of declining numbers of practitioners in mental health, recommendations are made for recruitment, academic and clinical education and practice.

A projected increase for occupational therapy personnel of 59.8% is forecast through 1990 ("OT Among," 1986) and the de-

Anne Hiller Scott is Clinical Assistant Professor, State University of New York, Health Science Center at Brooklyn, Occupational Therapy Program, Box 81, 450 Clarkson Avenue, Brooklyn, NY 11203.

The author would like to gratefully acknowledge Sharon Ezersky, Susan Haiman and Joyce Sabari for their thoughtful review and feedback.

mand for therapists currently exceeds the output of educational programs ("OT Shortages," 1989). However, decreasing numbers of therapists are pursuing positions in mental health creating a manpower crisis in this specialty area. The profession is mobilizing resources to develop broadly based strategies to reverse this trend and revitalize mental health practice (Baum, 1983; Bonder, 1987; Kolodner, Wiener & Frum, 1989). The intent of this article is to review literature from occupational therapy and other fields germane to specialty selection, reflect on critical issues for mental health practice and recommend viable approaches to stimulate renewal.

INTRODUCTION:
SPECIALIZATION OR WHAT'S IN A NAME

What is specialization and how do therapists classify their interventions? At any point in time how many therapists are practicing in a given specialty area? Although a critical point to the thesis of declining numbers in mental health is accurate documentation of shifts in personnel distribution, obtaining a representative census is not so straightforward. Before describing the distribution of therapists by specialty area, some caution is required due to overlap in definitions of specialty and differing approaches to classifying specialty areas.

Historical and longstanding distinctions acknowledged the areas of physical disabilities, mental health, gerontology and pediatrics. With the benefit of enabling legislation (Public Law 94-142), pediatrics has expanded considerably in the last decade to encompass 25% of practitioners. The American Occupational Therapy Association (AOTA) officially adopted special interest sections in 1978 and designated the areas of physical disabilities, mental health, developmental disabilities, gerontology and sensory integration. Recently the areas of administration and work programs have been added and new groups are forming in education, private practice and holistic practice. These classifications are not mutually exclusive and also represent different dimensions of categorization, e.g., age of patient (gerontology), type of disorder (mental or physical), age of onset of disorder (developmental disability), and type of intervention (sensory integration, work programs). For example, therapists often identify pediatrics as a specialty area and may be referring to working with children who have physical handicaps or developmental disabilities with sensory integration approaches. Some researchers have examined specialty preference as including mental health, physical disabilities, and pediatrics (Christie, Joyce & Moeller, 1985a), others used these categories and gerontology (Ezersky, Havazelet, Levenson, Scott & Zettler, 1985; Leonardelli & Caruso, 1986) or have used the AOTA designations of mental health, physical disabilities, developmental disabilities, gerontology and sensory integration (Swinehart & Wittman, 1988).

Specialty definition also raises concern regarding the holistic orientation of therapists. Breines (1986, 1987) suggested that the profession abandon specialty distinctions in favor of adopting an integrated identity and holistic approach to patients regardless of disability area. It is important to recognize the limitations of our current classification of specialty areas and advise future researchers to include relevant dimensions in analyzing specialty, such as type of disorder, age of patient, and even type of institutional setting to accurately capture salient characteristics of practice.

Little is known about how stable or fluid therapists are in their committment to practice in various specialty areas. There is a need to investigate tenure in specialty practice, occurrence and direction of shifts and factors which contribute to these shifts. There is some indication that as therapists move from their first to their second position, they leave practice in mental health and gerontology for positions in pediatrics and physical disabilities (Ezersky, Havazelet, Levenson, Scott & Zettler, 1985). Canadian researchers have begun to develop data regarding career patterns and influences contributing to changes of position (Madill, Brintnell, Stewin, Fitzsimmons & Macnab, 1985).

LITERATURE REVIEW

The following review includes studies relevant to specialty preference in occupational therapy and related health fields. Topics include specialty preference, personality characteristics, learning style, academic and clinical education, job satisfaction, and professional socialization.

Specialty Preference

The progressive decline of therapists practicing in mental health has persisted for more than a decade and is affecting the viability of this specialty area. Although the absolute numbers selecting mental health has not declined, the overall percentage of therapists specializing in mental health has decreased from 18% in 1973 to 8.5% in 1986 ("1986 Member," 1987). Cottrel (1987) has illustrated the corrosive impact of the declining number of practitioners (see Figure 1) reducing manpower resources, curtailing educational experiences for student training and reducing the availability of services for patients. Due to staffing shortages, mental health fieldwork experiences are among the most frequently cancelled compromising the potential for exposure to dynamic clinical sites (AOTA, 1987).

Personality Characteristics

How might personality characteristics contribute to favorable disposition towards various specialty areas? Brollier (1970) compared occupational therapists working in mental health and physical disabilities using the Edwards Personal Preference Scale. Occupational therapists working in physical disabilities were compared to physical therapists; and occupational therapists in mental health to social workers. The scores for each group of occupational therapists were similar to the professions to which they were matched. In addition, there were significant differences between occupational therapists in the two specialty areas. The mental health sample scored higher on dominance and autonomy; the physical disability group were lower on autonomy and deference and higher on order. The two groups were similar on variables of intraception, nurturance and achievement. It was concluded that differences in personality needs correlated with the different focuses in practice vis a vis content of practice, patient/therapist relationship and team interaction. Hendrickson (1962) studied a sample of psychiatric occupational therapists using the 16PF (16 Personality Factors) and also found high values on dominance and a related factor of being tough and self-reliant.

Figure 1

<u>Cycle Contributing to the Decline in the Number of Mental Health Occupational Therapy Practitioners</u>

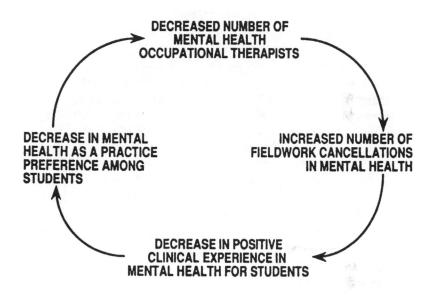

Note. From "Principles of Empirical Research" by Cottrell, R. F. (1987), unpublished paper, p. 4.

Learning Style

Stafford (1986) examined the influence of learning style on Level II Fieldwork Performance for physical disability and mental health experiences. The instruments used were the LSI (Learning Style Inventory) (Kolb, 1976, 1984) and the SOLAT (Your Style of Learning) (Torrance & Reynolds, 1980). A preference for active experimentation contributed positively to performance in each specialty area. In physical disabilities, scores were enhanced by a logical, sequential cognitive style, but these same qualities negatively affected some of the scores on the fieldwork performance instrument in mental health settings.

In nursing and medicine there has been some correspondence noted between learning style and specialty preference (Laschinger & Boss, 1984; Plovnick, 1975). Plovnick (1975) noted that medical students initial career preferences related to learning style and environmental factors, specifically courses and role models. Students who were more concrete learners as indicated by the LSI were more affected than others by the clinical work experience and attractive role models. Students selecting psychiatry demonstrated the divergent learning style incorporating use of concrete experience and reflective observation. Kolb (1981), the author of the LSI proposed that individuals chose fields that were compatible with their learning style and were further influenced and shaped by the learning norms of the profession. Occupational therapists fall within the accommodator learning style (Bennett, 1979) favoring concrete experience and active experimentation versus the use of reflective observation and abstract conceptualization.

Research suggests that learning style is a relevant variable impacting on specialty preference, academic and clinical education. Further study is warranted examining the relationship of learning styles of occupational therapy students and clinicians to specialty preference. If the concrete learning style does prevail, it follows that specialty choice may be more likely to be influenced by personal factors (role models and clinical experience) than by coursework, which would be the case for abstract learners.

Learning style would have strong relevance for how basic content is taught as well as how clinical fieldwork is integrated. Two studies noted dislike of academic coursework in mental health as a negative factor on specialty choice (Christie, Joyce & Moeller, 1985a; Ezersky, Havazelet, Levenson, Scott & Zettler, 1985). Feedback indicated that coursework was "... too nebulous, too general, too subjective, lacks empirical method, has no structure, is not concrete enough" (Christie, Joyce & Moeller, 1985a, p. 673). Burra and colleagues (1982) found that the attitudes of occupational therapy students became more negative following a psychiatry course. This finding was interpreted to be reflective of the absence of concomitant clinical exposure with the opportunity to see viable application of the field, rather than just exposure to theoretical material.

Page (1987) surveyed occupational therapy students rejecting mental health and identified five relevant areas: social stigma associated with the mentally ill, mental health course content, coupled with students cognitive level, dissatisfaction with practice setting (state hospital), and lack of previous experience or exposure. Page elaborated on the dualistic i.e., right or wrong quality of students' thinking style using Perry's (1969) developmental stages of ethical and cognitive development. "Students needing instructions, hierarchy and consistently right answers will have difficulty making meaning of multiple factors influencing disordered motivation, emotional response, or cognitive orientation" (Page, 1987, p. 2) of the mentally ill clinical population.

Schwartz (1984) has incorporated an approach to analyzing students' needs in clinical supervision utilizing Loevinger's (1977) developmental model of ego stages. The cognitive style at level 3 is characterized by conceptual simplicity and stereotypes, followed by multiplicity and then conceptual complexity. In this author's experience, students on Level I Fieldwork strongly identify with these descriptions as representative of their cognitive and affective reactions to the clinical experience. Schwartz offers guidelines as well for matching clinical instruction and supervision to the student's developmental level.

Findings regarding dislike of mental health coursework offer rich opportunity for speculation and further research. Potential studies could examine the relationship of cognitive style to course dislike, the presence, absence or timing of concomitant fieldwork on the integration of mental health content, factors related to the presentation and teaching methodologies employed, the influence of role models, previous exposure to psychiatric populations and attitudes toward the mentally ill.

Academic and Clinical Education

Swinehart & Wittman (1988) investigated specialty preference using AOTA specialty designations. Results indicated relatively minor shifts in specialty preference over the course of academic and clinical education. These findings suggest that specialty preference may be established and relatively firm prior to program admission. Although other investigators (Christie, Joyce & Moeller, 1985a; Ezersky, Havazelet, Scott & Zettler, 1989) have not had similar findings further research is warranted which tracks students' preferences on a longitudinal basis. One implication of this study is the need to actively recruit occupational therapy applicants attracted to mental health practice from the onset of their educational training.

Christie (1985a) and colleagues examined professional, academic and fieldwork influences on specialty. More than half (57%) of the sample indicated that their preference was not formed when they started the curriculum; 55% noted that their specialty interest developed or changed during fieldwork. The majority of respondents ranked the Level II Fieldwork experience as the primary influence on specialty choice. Smaller percentages, 20% and 16% respectively indicated preprofessional exposure and academic component as the highest ranking factors in their choice. The critical qualities of the fieldwork experience included the supervisor role model, communication/relationships, the attitudinal environment and variety in learning experiences and caseload. Effective supervision demonstrating the appropriate attitudinal and interpersonal variables was the most critical parameter of a positive clinical learning experience.

Christie and colleagues (1985b) elaborated on effective clinical teaching approaches and enumerated qualities of effective and ineffective supervisors. Interpersonal and communication skills, particularly in regard to giving feedback were primary problems for less effective supervisors who demonstrated a "constrictive supervision" pattern (Rosenblatt & Meyer, 1975). A developmental progression was noted among new supervisors who tended to be more controlling and concerned with their personal competencies as supervisory therapists. The authors recommended standardized training programs to prepare therapists for supervisory roles.

Although supervision was not confirmed as a primary factor by Ezersky, Havazelet, Scott & Zettler (1989), the affiliation experience, sense of effectiveness and influence of values, in addition to employment availability and specialty decision made prior to professional education were indicated as critical factors in specialty choice of recent occupational therapy graduates.

On exposure to fieldwork, 21% of occupational therapy students experienced intense emotional or personal responses such as depression, lack of confidence or anxiety which were dissuading factors from choosing a particular practice area (Christie, Joyce & Moeller, 1985a). In Mitchell's (1988) research, 53% of the students perceived the transition to Level II Fieldwork as stressful. There is related research for psychology interns on stressful events in training: poor quantity/quality of supervision, dealing with suicidal/acting out patients, narrow scope of learning experience and bureaucratic/political disputes (Cole, Kolko, & Craddick, 1981; Lerner, 1983). In a comparison of trainees and less experienced psychologists with more experienced clinicians, stress was moderated by years of experience and "felt competence level" (Lerner, 1983). The link between stress and competence has been implicated in studies of burnout among community mental health workers who cite feelings of inadequacy to perform tasks due to limited feedback, supervision or training (Cherniss & Egnatios, 1978; Pines, Aronson & Kafry, 1981; Pines & Maslach, 1978).

In regard to curriculum content, Christie (1985a) noted that limited emphasis and inadequate theoretical preparation contributed to students' avoidance of some specialty areas due to feelings of inadequacy and insecurity. Barris and Kielhofner (1986) have focused on the need for the profession to identify psychosocial coursework and skills relevant for practice. These authors comment that the eclecticism found in practice may contribute to the feeling that ". . . practice is nebulous and not clearly differentiated from other mental health professionals, a belief that might be reflected in the declining percentage of occupational therapists working in mental health" (Barris & Kielhofner, 1986, p. 535).

A study of fieldwork centers acknowledged as models for clinical training in mental health demonstrated a number of distinguishing characteristics (Kolodner, Wiener & Frum, 1989). Centers tended to have larger, multidisciplinary staff with greater numbers of occupational therapists. Supervisory education was offered to supervisors with expanded involvement encouraged in student training. Students participated in group seminars and were encouraged to self-evaluate their skills and performance. They were actively involved in generating referrals, evaluating, treating and reporting on interventions, and communicating with the multidisciplinary treatment team. Where ongoing research was being undertaken students were also offered exposure.

It should be acknowledged that there has been very little research on Level I Fieldwork specific to specialty preference. It is noteworthy however, that academic educators and fieldwork supervisors have a different emphasis on values and objectives for this experience than students (Kautzmann, 1987). Students primary emphasis was on clinical skills with lower rankings than clinical/academic faculty on: developing an awareness of the whole patient, overview of service delivery patterns, and opportunity for self-exploration and working out differences in the supervisory relationship. In addition, there is great variablility between schools regarding the scope and objectives of this clinical exposure (Leonardelli & Caruso, 1986).

Job Satisfaction

Burnout and lower work satisfaction has been noted for occupational therapists working in mental health (Brollier, Bender, Cyranowski & Velletri, 1986; Halperin, 1984; Sturgess & Poulsen, 1983). In reference to job satisfaction, Brollier (1985) found therapists employed in general hospital psychiatric settings had the lowest ratings. Brollier commented that dissatisfaction with pay and workload could be a source of burnout and withdrawal from the field. As students are exposed to many of these factors during the affiliation experience it is important to acknowledge their potential influence.

PROFESSIONAL SOCIALIZATION

How may some of the preceding findings on specialty preference be interpreted? Sabari (1985) has suggested that theories of professional socialization offer an important framework for understanding the educational process in occupational therapy. As a theoretical structure, professional socialization incorporates the characteristics of the individual and the cultural influences of the educational and clinical environment. The preexisting values, attitudes, skills and personality characteristics of students provide the matrix upon which academic and clinical education is superimposed.

Wentworth (1980) refers to the socialization process as one in which values, norms, roles and skills are acquired and internalized thus enabling the individual to function as a member of the cultural group. The socialization of a professional encompasses the following areas: (1) values and attitudes, (2) knowledge and skills, (3) behavior patterns and norms, and (4) development of a professional self-image through the process of internalizing and identifying with the new role (Becker, Geer, Hughes & Strauss, 1961; Sherlock & Morris, 1967; Wentworth, 1980). These processes span the period prior to recruitment, the predisposing anticipatory socialization through the academic phase, clinical training and acclimation to the job. Each phase may be characterized by value systems and orientations that influence learning and application of clinical skills or occupational knowledge.

Values represent the underlying beliefs which may support the individual's interest in distinct vocational pursuits (Katzell, 1964; Dawis & Lofquist, 1984). "Values are commands or directives for action" (Kramer, 1974, p. 29) to which individuals are committed. Images of the field or layman's conception of the nature of an occupation can serve to guide students in their early exploration of a field and expectations of the practice environment. Swinehart (1989) found that prior to acceptance in an occupational therapy program, students expressed a greater likelihood of working in physical disabilities than mental health.

What are the preconceived or naive images that potential recruits and beginning students have of occupational therapy? How many students view the field as primarily dealing with the physically handicapped? To what extent do their views incorporate the psychosocial perspective? How much are initial images of mental health practice strengthened or weakened over the course of classroom and clinical exposure? How well is the psychosocial content of practice integrated into the student's professional role identity? It is unsettling to consider that although all students are exposed to mental health coursework and the majority to psychosocial fieldwork so few elect to pursue practice in this area. The previously cited research findings regarding dislike of mental health coursework and fieldwork is suggestive of limited or inadequate integration of the psychosocial aspects of practice in the academic and clinical curriculum.

Sabari (1985) has commented on sources of inconsistencies between the content of professional socialization in the academic and clinical experiences in physical disabilities practice (Eliason & Gohl-Giese, 1979). Clinics expected students to be fluent in modalities that the school did not teach or support as part of the scope of practice. Sabari (1985) also recommended examination of whether students perceive incongruities between the mental health and physical disabilities faculty.

Burnett-Beaulieu (1982) has referred to the "fantasy image" of occupational therapy that motivates new recruits. Research indicates highly altruistic values of occupational therapy students (Madigan, 1985). To a great extent, the students' idealistic or layman's image of occupational therapy may be maintained during the academic education. However, clinical exposure confronts students and new therapists with a sense of loss and disenchantment with continual exposure to chronically ill and severely handicapped populations in often nonsupportive work environments (Burnett-Beaulieu, 1982). The sociological literature in nursing on professional socialization and reality shock (Kramer, 1974) provides some conceptual understanding of this phenomenon, which may also have relevance for attraction to specialty areas.

Nursing

In nursing, the period of transition to the clinic or workplace has been observed to generate intense anxiety and shock due to the disparity and disjunction between the academic and clinical experience (Kramer, 1974). Kramer (1974) coined the term "reality shock" to refer to "the discrepant, shock like reactions that follow when the aspirant professional perceives that many professional ideals and values are not operationalized and go unrewarded in the work setting" (p. vii). Conflict emerges between the professional values of the school and the bureaucratic values of the organization. The experience of new graduates is compared to culture shock. The outcome of this confrontation can be growth producing conflict resolution and adoption of professional and/or bureaucratic goals or a sense of role deprivation. If situational constraints severely limit role enactment, extreme dissatisfaction can result in exodus from the field.

In developing a thesis of professional socialization, Kramer (1974) analyzed common conflicts of new nurses: the professional-bureaucratic influence, difference between explicit expectations of the school and implicit expectations of the work environment, difference between the cosmopolitan or professional orientation and the localistic perspectives of work, in addition to individualistic concerns.

Concerns of nurses were: clinical uncertainty, competency gap, constancy of time pressure and time orientation, sociocultural differences between institutions and racial conflicts as they affected work performance. Limited perception of competency was a serious problem. In the work environment, competency in manual/technical skills was more highly emphasized, whereas new nurses identified with the psychosocial aspects of nursing. Confusion around role definition, lack of competency, particularly in interpersonal relationships contributed to undermining the new professional's confidence and effectiveness. Difficulty in interpersonal relationships was cited in relation to interactions with supervisors and staff (not in relation to dealing with patients). Limited skill in interpersonal competency contributed to difficulty for nursing students in negotiating within the system to diminish reality shock and facilitate role integration. Although nurses have nurturing values predisposing them to service, they scored low on measures of empathy (LaMonica, 1974; LaMonica & Karshmer, 1978), and therefore were at a disadvantage in accurately perceiving the bureaucratic perspective and becoming effective change agents in dealing with supervisors and co-workers.

Of major relevance in the socialization process was the development of self-concept as a nurse. Kramer and Schmalenberg (1978) outlined the following aspects as central to nurses level of self-esteem: (1) living up to one's values and aspirations, (2) experiencing success and competence in valued areas, (3) receiving acceptance, respect and concerned treatment from significant others. Levels of self-confidence were undermined in the clinical setting by lack of clarity regarding roles and sense of inadequacy in performing skills, coupled with limited positive feedback from others.

Measures suggested to enhance self-esteem included assessment of new graduates skills with opportunities to practice them, regular feedback from a consistent supervisory figure and more realistic preparation in school. The development of self-evaluation and self-reinforcement techniques was also encouraged when feedback was not available in the work environment. In addition, more recognition on the job for the psychosocial and teaching aspects of nursing care was advocated as well as preparation of supervisory staff to work with new graduates.

To address the discrepancy between school and work subcultures and to help the professional nurse develop a bicultural stance; Kramer and Schmalenberg (1978) developed two programs, a reality shock program for new graduates and an anticipatory socialization program to prepare student nurses for the stresses and conflicts they would encounter upon entering the clinical setting. The major obstacles for new graduates were the differences between the real world and laboratory environment structured by the school and the artificial rather self-sealing theories that students were taught. The authors maintained that professional practice was characterized by development of effective theories for practice. This included elements of diagnosis, hypothesis development/testing, and the notion of personal causation. Personal causation was defined as "performing responsibly under conditions of the real world—stress, under pressure of deadlines, constrained by time and money" (Kramer & Schmalenberg, 1978, p. 108). In implementing one's theory of practice, the integration of the dimensions of technical and interpersonal components were assumed. Values were seen as vehicles which shape one's approach in the development of theories for practice.

Psychiatry

Bucher and Strauss (1961) identified a "process" model for studying professions and specialization. Groupings which emerge from within a profession are known as "segments." Specialties are major segments within a profession and close examination can reveal differences in identity, values, role definition and interests. Bucher and Stelling (1977) maintain that assumption of a specialization is a turning point in which one develops further differentiation in professional identity. In addition, the character of the socialization experience can be expected to vary between segments of a specialty and those differences can effect qualities sought in recruits, the content of appropriate experience and learning, and influence what perspectives are seen as critical.

Many occupations are characterized by a "core act" (Bucher & Strauss, 1961; Bucher & Stelling, 1977) a distinguishing feature of practice that relates to the nature and definition of the work. For psychoanalytically oriented psychiatrists, it was the process of the interpersonal interaction with the patient in the course of the psychotherapy or psychoanalysis. This integral and central activity is in contrast to the core acts of many other specialty areas, e.g., surgery, obstetrics or internal medicine. In medicine, psychiatry is a segment or specialty which conforms poorly to the prevailing structure of the medical school curriculum and typical patterns of practice. It is noteworthy for example, that even psychiatric residents felt they used their medical skills less than 75% of the time (Taintor, 1983).

A critical study of the socialization of psychiatric residents also revealed major difficulty and discomfort in adjusting to the clinical training site (Bucher, Stelling & Dommeruth, 1969; Bucher & Stelling, 1977). Similar to findings for nurses, an intense period of initial anxiety or confusion was noted for psychiatric residents, who took six months to a year to fully adjust. The sense of competence and physician's identity gained in previous internships did not help ease the transition to the training program. One of the supervising psychiatrists indicated that the initial adjustment involved "confronting complex, deep (unconscious) and extremely disturbing emotions, first in the patients and then in themselves, as interactions with patients arouses similar complimentary emotions in residents" (Bucher & Stelling, 1977, p. 193).

Bucher and Stelling (1977) maintained that professional socialization resulted mostly from the impact of the structural and situational aspects of the training program. The major elements of the socialization process were: self and others, role models and self-evaluation, development and mastery. The authors saw increasing mastery linked to beginning acquisition of professional identity, commitment and clearer conceptions of career directions. "The sense of mastery is a very important component in feeling that one is in the right place . . . [there] must be some validation of role performance in order for people to continue to perform particular roles" (Bucher & Stelling, 1977, 211-212).

Role definitions, scope of practice and specialized interpersonal skills necessary for patient treatment and team leadership roles were not mastered sufficiently in the academic curriculum of the psychiatric residents. The preceding material is presented to substantiate the assumption that the socialization process can vary by area of specialization and that psychiatry in particular may offer differing socialization experiences.

To what extent is there consensus about the core act of occupational therapy? The use of activities is debated and values related to occupation vary in treatment settings and practice areas. Occupational role or role enactment is dependent upon satisfactory mastery of knowledge and skills, in concert with congruent role orientations and values of the student, the school, the profession and the training/employing institution. Sabari (1985) has suggested that increasing consistency between the academic and clinical elements of occupational therapy education will strengthen the outcome of professional socialization. Ambiguity, difficulty in defining roles and conflict in implementing one's role expectations can relate to differences in values, deficiencies in skills and lack of grounding in negotiating within the system.

REFLECTIONS

What are the parallels between the experiences of nurses and psychiatric residents with professional socialization and occupational therapy students? Do occupational therapy students become disenchanted with the field? Nordholm and Westbrook (1981) found that Australian occupational therapy students indicated the highest likelihood of leaving the profession compared to several other allied health groups. These students also expressed the greatest amount of change in their conception of the field (layman's image) with there being greater emphasis on both the psychosocial and biological content and less on crafts.

Do occupational therapy students experience stress and discontinuity between the academic and clinical training? There is strong evidence that occupational therapy students find the transition to clinical fieldwork stressful (Christie, Joyce & Moeller, 1985a; Mitchell, 1988). A major stress or support is the supervisor and her or his qualities as a role model and effectiveness in creating a supportive interpersonal climate (Christie, Joyce & Moeller, 1985b). Sense of effectiveness or competence is a critical variable contributing to specialty preference (Ezersky, Havazelet, Scott, & Zettler, 1989), which can reduce role stress and strengthen role identity.

Do occupational therapy students and practitioners experience conflicts in value orientations? In a study of clinical reasoning in physical disabilities practice, Fleming (1988) encountered a value conflict between the scientific and humanitarian orientation to practice. For some therapists the technique was viewed as the primary therapy, for others the interpersonal elements of the patient-therapist interaction were included. "All therapists felt that understanding patients as people was not a reimbursable service . . ." (Fleming, 1988, p. 5) and this element of practice was not documented. This presented a dilemma and strong conflict for therapists in the medical setting.

Johnson (1977) has commented on the dichotomy between our humanitarian and nurturing values and the opposing qualities needed in the work place to deal with power, politics and confrontation. Yerxa (1979) describes the conflict between our supportive-giving orientation to patients and the controlling-directing qualities needed to promote professional autonomy and status. She concludes that "the conflict between these two sets of values create considerable ambivalence, frustration and professional schizophrenia" (Yerxa, 1978, p. 28). These concerns appear consistent with Madigan's (1985) findings using a work values instrument. Students' highest value was altruism and the next to lowest was management. This would have direct implications for skills in leadership. It seems important to note, as well, Brollier's (1970) finding that therapists in mental health ranked higher on autonomy and dominance.

Do occupational therapists have difficulty negotiating the transition from student to therapist? A study of perceived problems of beginning occupational therapists mirrors those of neophyte nurses with reality shock. The most powerful problems were time management and pressure, effective authority/collaboration particularly in conveying the role of occupational therapy, and competence/confidence (Allen & Cruickshank, 1977). These authors suggested that beginning therapists are: (1) not successful in explaining their diverse roles, (2) insecure regarding their skills and therefore have difficulty in being assertive in explaining their roles and (3) find themselves in alien systems without enough knowledge of how to evaluate systems and work effectively within them. Concern was also expressed regarding the non-assertive characteristics of most occupational therapy students.

Relating some of the findings on professional socialization and learning style to occupational therapy, it is hypothesized that the role identity of the specialty areas of mental health and physical disabilities incorporate different "core acts." The occupational knowledge base differs for physical disabilities and mental health and curriculums' basic emphasis may be more focused on physical disabilities theory and technique. In mental health, furthermore, there is a greater emphasis on interpersonal relationships and the affective domain which can be difficult to teach and evaluate effectively. As in nursing, students probably have predominantly nurturing and service values, with limited exposure to enhancing empathy and developing bureaucratic problem solving skills. In addition, the students' learning style could be more compatible with the concrete learning required for physical disabilities interventions. There may also be greater discrepancies between theories and interventions presented in the academic and clinical components of mental health practice. Generally, there is more role blurring and lack of clarity regarding role definition in mental health, particularly in large state hospitals with heavily bureaucratic structures. Due to these factors, occupational therapy students may be more likely to experience reality shock in mental health settings and find this area less attractive supported by a sense of limited competency and inadequate academic preparation.

RECOMMENDATIONS

Any suggestions for enhancing education in psychosocial occupational therapy and increasing the numbers of practitioners must acknowledge broad demographic, social and political forces germane to this problem. Recommendations will be made here for recruitment, academic and clinical education and practice.

Recruitment

Where will the new therapists come from? There is a decline in the number of college age students and concomitantly women are pursuing broader career options. The annual number of new occupational therapy graduates has been a relatively stable 2,300 for the last several years, with no significant increase in applicants ("OT Shortages," 1989). Recruitment efforts must be a priority and aggressive strategies are required. It will not be enough for occupational therapy schools and AOTA to spearhead these activities; all therapists and departments need to be involved. As an innovative approach to combatting chronic staff shortages more hospitals and institutions are offering students scholarships for service commitments upon graduation. The New York State Health Service Corps, for example provides scholarships to occupational therapy students for service commitments in state hospital and voluntary institutions.

To attract students effective publicity resources and expanded opportunity for open house visits, volunteer work, work-study and cooperative education programs are needed. Outreach to appropriate high school and college groups is necessary. Identification of individuals who would be favorably predisposed to working with the mentally ill is critical. Psychology majors and those interested in social service may be approached through clubs, service organizations and interested faculty at most colleges and universities.

Academic Programs

Admission criteria are the portals of the profession and recruits are the raw material of future specialty choice. Sabari (1985) has suggested that programs clarify the qualities they value in recruits.

In academic programs, the recruitment process and curriculum content needs to focus on attitudes, values and personality characteristics which shape the complexion of our future professionals and impact on specialty choice. Recent research suggests differences between occupational therapy, physical therapy and speech pathology students on measures of values and implications for resultant career choice and education (Madill, Macnab & Brintnell, 1989). There is a need for identification of critical variables such as empathy that will support and nurture interest in the mentally ill as well as strengthen one's professional armamentarium. A related question is how effective is the curriculum in significantly changing attitudes and values? Studies of medical students and graduate students in health programs suggest that modification, if possible is not long lived (Feldman & Crook, 1984; Markham, 1979; Rezler & Flaherty, 1985). If this is also the case for occupational therapy, programs will need to seek individuals who already manifest the desired qualities.

In relation to curricula organization, Breines (1987) recommends organizing coursework to reinforce our common philosophical values and professional identity. It is important to emphasize the generic and integrating qualities of occupational therapy values and content across specialty areas. This encourages a truly holistic approach to patients regardless of type of disability. Bing (1986) espouses underpinning education with fundamental historical values and beliefs commenting that a technological focus is "but shifting sand" (p. 24). The dialogue generated by Leonardelli and Gratz (1986) on the purpose of professional schools regarding the integration of technical competency with problem solving abilities is apropos. The Task Force on Target Populations (1974) forewarned that:

> if occupational therapy is to survive as a profession, the schisms within the profession related to diagnostic or disability entities need to be removed by focusing on the essence of occupational therapy rather than a disability or pathological orientation. (p. 158)

The psychosocial content and teaching methodologies must be scrutinized to foster a better match between students' cognitive styles and capacity to relate to this area positively and effectively. Appreciating the role of theory in guiding practice is critical. Helping students develop a sense of mastery through guided application of theoretical models is essential. Spencer (1986) identified the primary components of psychosocial occupational therapy in education as interpersonal learning through interaction with experienced therapists, staff and patients and exploration of value commitments. Hansen (1986) recommends closer scrutiny of teaching techniques and the effectiveness of values education. Increased exposure to effective clinical role models in the classroom can also help. In the clinical fieldwork, structured learning is important to promote realistic expectations and sense of mastery with the psychiatric population. The clinical reasoning process needs to be unraveled so that students can make it more tangible. Cohen (1989) and Niestadt (1987) offer suggestions for enhancing students clinical reasoning skills.

Students need to be prepared for the powerful emotional experiences of clinical fieldwork. The discontinuity between class and clinic has been documented in medicine and nursing. Target 2000 (1986) has recommended planned "integrating experiences during and after the fieldwork" (p. 95). Fostering more consistency between the academic and clinical content would go far in reducing the impact of reality shock. Introducing models such as Kramer & Schmalenberg's (1978) reality shock and anticipatory socialization programs would offer innovative and viable approaches to help students identify value conflicts, and effective problem solving strategies.

The area where the most promise or peril exists for reversing or engaging specialty interests is the fieldwork experience. If, as the sociological literature implies for nursing, the clinical experience is the most powerful socializing agent, the greatest challenge is borne by the clinical educator. The technical aspects of practice, as well as the interpersonal and affective components need to be orchestrated by the supervisor to promote the synthesis of clear role identity, sound skills and strong professional commitment in the beginning therapist. Nowhere are the educational and supervisory skills of the individual therapist more critical. Perhaps a weak link in the system is the expectation that the therapist with one year of practice has the experience, knowledge base and resources to effect this professional transformation in the neophyte therapist. Students are vulnerable and impressionable. The successes, as well as the inevitable disappointments and disillusionment of the clinical exposure is a palpable and painful reality, which hopefully can be used to promote growth rather than flight.

How can we prepare and equip supervising therapists for this most important professional trust? Several models that account for the developmental nature of this process are available (Burnett-Beaulieu, 1982; Crist, 1986; Frum & Opacich, 1987; Pelland, 1987; Schwartz, 1984). In addition developing skills that accommodate for both the student and the clinical educator's cognitive levels and learning style is paramount. Geyer (1988), for example has outlined the application of Kolb's Learning Style to clinical supervision. A more standardized approach to developing supervisory skills has been advocated and should be pursued (Huss, 1984; Christie, Joyce & Moeller, 1985b). The study of Model Fieldwork Centers is valuable in identifying ways to enhance clinical experience in mental health and resource materials available for therapists' use (Kolodner, Wiener, Frum, 1989). Developing supervisory skills is a sound professional investment. Research indicates that leadership and supervisory qualities of the occupational therapy chief were key in the "degree of satisfaction and level of commitment experienced by staff therapists" (Madill, Brintnell, Stewin, Fitzsimmons & Macnab, 1986, p. 94).

Johnson has commented on therapists' belief that the educational system can resolve problems, avoiding recognition of the need to change practice patterns. In mental health we need to examine the viability of current models of practice with various populations, such as the acute short-term population, the chronic deinstitutionalized population, etc. (Denton, 1986; Jackson, 1984; Kaplan, 1984; Short, 1984). We have not moved with the patient into the community and this may reflect inadequate practice models (Bonder, 1987). Goldenberg and Quinn (1984) document a successful example of providing home care to the mentally ill in the community. Johnson's (1983) recommendations for practice models viable in today's consumer and medical marketplace should be considered. Occupational therapists have been able to make a major impact on service needs in the school system. However, we who have some of the most valuable professional skills to offer the deinstitutionalized mentally ill have not yet made such an impact on the community mental health system.

One pressing reality of our labor pool is that our membership is 96% female. To what extent does the job market accommodate to the multiple role demands of professional women. The impact of multiple role commitments is a major influence on career patterns (Madill, Brintnell, Stewin, Fitzsimmons & Macnab, 1985). Perhaps the flexible scheduling of contract work and pediatric practice is an incentive that employers in mental health need to consider to recruit and retain therapists. Berman (1988) offers a number of creative strategies to attract and retain qualified practitioners in mental health.

Many fruitful areas for research need to be tilled in the future: values, learning styles, interpersonal skill development, empathy, supervision, role modeling, development of mastery and competence and the evolution of clinical reasoning. A final recommendation, informed by the rich and compelling material from the sociological studies in other fields is a call for qualitative research on students, beginning therapists and new and experienced supervisors in mental health practice. This will provide a critical perspective on the "reality shock" and "fantasy images" of our practice. To move from these fantasies to a more favorable reality will require our collective energies, strategies and activities; however, facilitating problem-solving and promoting a more functional adaptation to the current environmental needs should be familiar to us—isn't this what we do so well in our every day practice?

REFERENCES

Allen, A. S., & Cruickshank, D. R. (1977). Perceived problems of occupational therapists. A subset of the professional curriculum. *American Journal of Occupational Therapy*, *31*(9), 557-564.

American Occupational Therapy Association. (1987). *1987 Education data survey final report*. Rockville, MD: American Occupational Therapy Association.

Barris, R., & Kielfhofner, G. (1986). Beliefs, perspectives, and activities of psychosocial occupational therapy educators. *American Journal of Occupational Therapy*, *40*(8), 535-541.

Baum, C. D. (1983). Strategic integrated management system – SIMS. *American Journal of Occupational Therapy*, *37*(9), 595-600.

Becker, H. S., Geer, B., Hughes, E. C., & Strauss, A. L. (1961) *Boys in white: Student culture in medical school*. Chicago: University of Chicago Press.

Bennett, N. (1979). *Learning style of health professions compared to preference for continuing education format*. Unpublished doctoral dissertation. University of Illinois: Chicago.

Berman, C. R. (1988). Recruitment and retention: Approaches that work. In, *Acute care psychiatry. Practical strategies and collaborative approaches*. Rockville, MD: American Occupational Therapy Association.

Bing, R. (1986). Perspectives on the values underlying occupational therapy practice. In, *Occupational therapy education: Target 2000* (pp. 21-24). Rockville, MD: American Occupational Therapy Association.

Bonder, B. R. (1987). Occupational therapy in mental health: Crisis or opportunity? *American Journal of Occupational Therapy*, *41*(8), 495-499.

Breines, E. (1986). *Origins and adaptations: A philosophy of practice*. Lebanon, NJ: Geri-Rehab.

Breines, E. (1987). Pragmatism as a foundation for occupational therapy curricula. *American Journal of Occupational Therapy*, *41*(8), 522-525.

Brollier, C. (1970). Personality characteristics of three allied health professional groups. *American Journal of Occupational Therapy*, *24*(7), 500-505.

Brollier, C. (1985). A multivariate predictive study of staff OTR's job satisfaction: Some results of importance to psychosocial occupational therapy. *Occupational Therapy in Mental Health*, *5*, 13-28.

Brollier, C., Bender, D., Cyranowski, J., & Velletri, C. M. (1986). A pilot study among hospital based occupational therapists. *Occupational Therapy in Mental Health*, *6*(5), 285-299.

Bucher, R., & Strauss, A. (1961). Professions in process. *American Journal of Sociology*, *66*, 325-334.

Bucher, R., Stelling, R. J., & Dommermuth, P. (1969). Implications of prior socialization for residency programs in psychiatry. *Archives of General Psychiatry*, *20*, 395-407.

Bucher, R., & Stelling, R. J. (1977). *Becoming professsional*. Beverly Hills: Sage.

Burnett-Beaulieu, S. (1982). Occupational therapy profession dropouts: Escape from the grief process. *Occupational Therapy in Mental Health*, *2*(2), 45.

Burra, P., Kalin, P., Leichner, P., Waldron, J. J., Handforth, J. R., Jarrett, F. J., & Amarai, B. (1982). The ATP-30 – A scale for measuring medical students attitudes toward psychiatry. *Medical Education*, *16*, 31-38.

Cherniss, C. (1980). *Professional burnout in human service organizations*. NY: Praeger.

Cherniss, C., & Egnatios, E. (1978). Is there job satisfaction in community mental health? *Community Mental Health Journal*, *14*(4), 309-318.

Christie, B., Joyce, P., & Moeller, P. (1985a). Fieldwork experience, part I:

Impact on practice preference. *American Journal of Occupational Therapy*, *39*(10), 671-674.

Christie, B., Joyce, P., & Moeller, P. (1985b). Fieldwork experience, part II: The supervisor's dilemma. *American Journal of Occupational Therapy*, *39*(10), 675-681.

Cohen, E. (1989). Fieldwork education: Shaping a foundation for clinical reasoning. *American Journal of Occupational Therapy*, *43*(4), 240-244.

Cole, M. A., Kolko, D. J., & Craddick, R. A. (1981). The quality and process of internship experiences. *Professional Psychology*, *12*(5), 570-577.

Cottrell, R. F. (1987). *Principles of empirical research*. Unpublished paper, New York University, Department of Occupational Therapy, New York, NY.

Crist, P. H. (1986). *Contemporary issues in clinical education*. Thorofare, NJ: Slack.

Dawis, R. V., & Lofquist, L. H. (1984). *A psychological theory of work adjustment. An individual differences model and its applications*. Minneapolis, MN: University of Minnesota Press.

Denton, P. (1986). Occupational therapy practice in acute care: Changes, challenges, and coping strategies. *Mental Health Special Interest Section Newsletter*, *9*(1), pp. 1, 3-4.

Eliason, M., & Gohl-Giese, A. (1979). A question of professional boundaries: Implications for educational programs. *American Journal of Occupational Therapy*, *33*, 175-179.

Ezersky, S., Havazelet, L., Levenson, F., Scott, A., & Zettler, C. (1985). Factors affecting specialty selection of recent graduates. *Proceedings of American Occupational Therapy Association Program Director's Fall Meeting, Scottsdale, AZ* (pp. 1-21). Rockville, MD: American Occupational Therapy Association.

Ezersky, S., Havazelet, L., Scott, A., & Zettler, C. (1989) Specialty preference in occupational therapy. *American Journal of Occupational Therapy*, *43*(4), 227-233.

Feldman, E., & Crook, J. (1985). Personal characteristics of health professionals. Can they be changed by an educational program? *Journal of Allied Health*, *13*(3), 163-168.

Fleming, M. H. (1988). The therapist with the three track mind. *Mini course in clinical reasoning*, (pp. 1-22). Rockville, MD: American Occupational Therapy Foundation.

Frum, D., & Opacich, K. (1987). *Supervision. Development of professional competence*. Rockville, MD: American Occupational Therapy Association.

Geyer, L. A. (1988, July 11). Affiliation supervision requires knowledge of learning styles. *O.T. Advance*, pp. 10-12, 14.

Goldenberg, K., & Quinn, B. (1985). Community occupational therapy associates: A model of private practice for community occupational therapy. *Occupational Therapy in Health Care*, *2*(2), 15-23.

Halperin, I. (1984). *The "burnout" syndrome within three specialty areas of occupational therapy: Causes, characteristics and implications*. Unpublished master's thesis, New York University, New York: NY.

Hansen, R. A. (1986). Occupational therapy values education. In, *Occupational therapy education: Target 2000* (pp. 19-21). Rockville, MD: American Occupational Therapy Association.

Hendrickson, D. (1962). Personality variables. Significant departures of occupational therapists from population norms. *American Journal of Occupational Therapy, 16*(3), 127-130.

Huss, J. (1984). Whither thou goest. *American Journal of Occupational Therapy, 38*(2), 81-83.

Jackson, G. A. (1984). Short-term psychiatric treatment: How will occupational therapy adapt? *Occupational Therapy Journal of Mental Health, 4*, 11-17.

Johnson, J. (1977). Humanitarianism and accountability: A challenge for occupational therapy on its 60th anniversary. *American Journal of Occupational Therapy, 31*(10), 631-637.

Johnson, J. (1983). The changing medical marketplace as a context for the practice of occupational therapy. In, *Health Through Occupation*, Ed. G. Kielhofner, pp. 163-177. Philadelphia: F. A. Davis.

Kaplan, K. (1984). Introduction: Short term treatment in occupational therapy. *Occupational Therapy Journal of Mental Health, 4*(3), 5-9.

Katzell, R. A. (1964). Personal values, job satisfaction and job behavior. In H. Borow (Ed.), Man in a world at work. Boston, MA: Houghton Mifflin.

Kautzmann, L. (1987). Perceptions of the purpose of the level I fieldwork. *American Journal of Occupational Therapy, 41*(9), 595-600.

Kolb, D. A. (1976). *Learning style inventory: Technical Manual*. Boston: McBer & Co.

Kolb, D. (1984). *Experiential learning*. Englewood Cliffs, NJ: Prentice-Hall.

Kolodner, E. L., Wiener, W. J., & Frum, D. (1989). *Models for Mental Health Fieldwork*. Rockville, MD: American Occupational Therapy Association.

Kramer, M. (1974). *Reality shock: Why nurses leave nursing*. C. V. Mosby.

Kramer, M., & Schmalenberg, C. (1977). *Path to biculturalism*. Wakefield, MA: Contemporary.

LaMonica, E. (1974). Empathy training as a major thrust of a staff development program. *Journal of Nursing Education, 17*(2), 3-11.

LaMonica, E., & Karshmer, J. (1978). Empathy: Educating nurses in professional practice. *Journal of Nursing Education, 17*(2), 3-11.

Laschinger, H. K. & Boss, M. W. (1984) Learning styles of nursing students and career choices. *Journal of Advanced Nursing, 9*, 375-380.

Leonardelli, C. A., & Caruso, L. A. (1986). Level I fieldwork: Issues and needs. *American Journal of Occupational Therapy, 40* (4), 258-264.

Leonardelli, C. A., & Gratz, R. R. (1986). Occupational therapy education: The relationship of purpose, objectives, and teaching models. *American Journal of Occupational Therapy, 40*(2), 96-102.

Lerner, J. R. (1983). *Correlates of reported stress in professional situations: A study of trainees and graduates in a counseling psychology program*. Unpublished doctoral dissertation. University of Pennsylvania: PA.

Loevinger, J. (1977). *Ego development: Conceptions and theories*. San Francisco: Jossey Bass.

Madigan, M. J. (1985). Characteristics of students in occupational therapy education programs. *American Journal of Occupational Therapy, 39*(1), 41-48.

Madill, H. M., Brintnell, E. S. G., Stewin, L. L., Fitzsimmons, G. W., & Macnab, D. (1985). Career patterns in two groups of Alberta occupational therapists. *Canadian Journal of Occupational Therapy, 52*(4), 195-201.

Madill, H. M., Brintnell, E. S. G., Stewin, L. L., Fitzsimmons, G. W., & Macnab, D. (1986). Occupational therapy career patterns in profile. *Canadian Journal of Occupational Therapy, 53*(2), 86-95.

Madill, H. M. , Macnab, D., & Brintnell, E. S. G. (1989 In Press). Student values and preferences: What do they tell us about programme selection?. *Canadian Journal of Occupational Therapy*.

Markham, B. (1979). Can a behavioral science course change medical students attitudes? *Journal of Psychiatric Education, 3*, 44-54.

Mitchell, M. (1988). *Coping strategies associated with the transition from academic learning to clinical internship: A pilot study*. Great Southern Occupational Therapy Conference. Orlando: FL.

Niestadt, M. E. (1987). Classroom as clinic: A model for teaching clinical reasoning in occupational therapy education. *American Journal of Occupational Therapy, 41*(10), 631-637.

1986 member data survey: Summary report. (1987, September). *Occupational Therapy News*, pp. 11-13.

Nordholm, L. A. & Westbrook, M. T. (1981). Career selection, satisfaction and aspirations among students in five health professions. *Australian Psychologist, 16*, 63-76.

OT among the twenty fastest growing occupations. (1986). *Dataline 1982-1985*, (p. 24). Rockville, MD: American Occupational Therapy Association.

OT Shortages continue. (1989, January). *Occupational Therapy News*. pp. 20-21.

Page, M. S. (1987). Factors that influence students choice of mental health as a career. *Mental Health Special Interest Section Newsletter, 10*(3), 1-3.

Pelland, M. J. (1987). A conceptual model for the instruction and supervision of treatment planning. *American Journal of Occupational Therapy, 41*(6), 351-359.

Perry, W. G. (1970). Forms of intellectual and cognitive development in the college years. NY: Holt, Rinehart & Winston.

Pines, A. M., Aronson, E. & Kafry, D. (1981). *Burnout: From tedium to personal growth*. NY: Macmillan.

Pines, A. M., & Maslach, C. (1978). Characteristics of staff burnout in mental health settings. *Hospital and Community Psychiatry, 29*(4), 233-237.

Plovnick, M. (1975). Primary care career choices and medical student learning styles. *Journal of Medical Education, 50*, 845-855.

Rezler, A. G., & Flaherty, J. (1985). *Interpersonal dimensions in medical education*. NY: Springer.

Rosenblatt, A., & Meyer, J. F. (1975). Objectionable supervisory styles: Student views. *Social Work, 20,* 184-189.

Sabari, J. (1985). Professional socialization: Implications for occupational therapy education. *American Journal of Occupational Therapy, 39,* 96-102.

Schwartz, K. B. (1984). An approach to supervision of students on fieldwork. *American Journal of Occupational Therapy, 38*(6), 393-397.

Sherlock, B. J., & Morris, R. (1967). The evolution of the professional: A Paradigm. *Sociological Inquiries, 37,* 27-46.

Short, J. E. (1984). Changing role expectations of psychiatric occupational therapists. *Occupational Therapy Journal of Mental Health,* 19-27.

Spencer, J, C. (1986). Perceptions of a recent graduate. A broad activity analysis of occupational therapy education. *Occupational therapy education. Target 2000.* Rockville, MD: American Occupational Therapy Association.

Stafford, E. M. (1986). Relationship between occupational therapy student learning styles and clinic performance. *American Journal of Occupational Therapy, 40*(1), 34-39.

Sturgess, J., & Poulsen, A. (1983). The prevalence of burnout in occupational therapists. *Occupational Therapy in Mental Health, 3*(4), 47-60.

Swinehart, S. (1989). *Are admission procedures biased toward certain practice preferences?* Poster Session presented at Annual Conference of the American Occupational Therapy Association. Baltimore, MD.

Swinehart, S., & Wittman, P. (1988). *Variables affecting specialty choice in occupational therapy practice.* Paper presented at Annual Conference of the American Occupational Therapy Association. Phoenix, AZ.

Taintor, Z., Murphy, M., Seiden, X., & Val, E. (1983). Psychiatric residency training: Relationship and value development. *American Journal of Psychiatry, 140*: 778-780.

Task Force on Target Populations. (1974). *American Journal of Occupational Therapy, 28*(3), 158-163.

Torrance E. P., & Reynolds, C: (1980). *Norms – Technical Manual for Your Style of Learning and Thinking – Form C.* Athens: GA, University of Georgia, Department of Educational Psychology.

Wentworth, W. (1980). *Context and Understanding – An Inquiry into Socialization Theory.* NY: Elsevier.

Yerxa, E. (1978). The philosophical base of occupational therapy. In, *Occupational therapy: 2001 AD.* pp. 26-30. American Occupational Therapy Association.

Enriching the Fieldwork II Experience: A Recruitment Strategy for Psychosocial Occupational Therapy

Elisabeth Winnie Ebb, MS, OTR/L
Susan Haiman, MPS, OTR/L

SUMMARY. The shortage of occupational therapists working in mental health is of serious concern to the profession. This article will briefly describe the current issues related to manpower, recruitment and level II fieldwork education. It will then discuss the development, utilization and impact of one educational program designed to increase student interest in mental health by supplementation of the level II fieldwork experience. In conclusion, this paper will give suggestions for future strategies that may lead to both improved level II education and increased student interest in mental health as a career choice.

Currently, much attention is being focused on the severe manpower shortage in occupational therapy. This shortage seems to be related to a decreasing number of college age students, a leveling off of students graduating from accredited occupational therapy

Elisabeth Winnie Ebb is Senior Occupational Therapist/Student Coordinator at the Payne Whitney Clinic, New York Hospital-Cornell Medical Center, 525 East 68th Street, New York, NY 10021.

Susan Haiman is Assistant Director, Department of Therapeutic Activities, Payne Whitney Clinic, New York Hospital-Cornell Medical Center; and Lecturer, Department of Psychiatry, Cornell Medical College.

The authors would like to thank the following people; Gail Fidler, OTR, FAOTA; Susan B. Fine, MA, OTR/L, FAOTA; Mark Rosenfeld, PhD, OTR/L; Arlene Michaelson Baily, MS, OTR/L, CRC; Tina Barth, MA, OTR/L, CRC; Dawn Beverly, OTR/L; Joan Feder, MA, OTR/L; Ellen Rabinowitz, MPS, OTR/L; Nadine Revheim, MS, OTR/L; Perri Schwimmer Stern, MA, OTR/L; and the staff of the Payne Whitney Clinic Therapeutic Activities Department.

programs, difficulty attracting minority or nontraditional students to the profession and limited public knowledge about occupational therapy as a viable career choice. In mental health this manpower shortage has been even more acute as only a small percentage of occupational therapy graduates are choosing psychiatry as their area of specialization. At present there are many exciting recruitment strategies being explored to increase the general pool of students entering occupational therapy educational programs. Less attention has been paid to ways in which the profession might influence a larger number of todays graduating students to choose mental health as their area of career specialization. Evidence suggests that a critical factor in influencing students' choice of specialization is the supervisory relationship during the level II fieldwork experience. Therefore, this supervisory experience represents a potentially critical opportunity for the recruitment of psychosocial occupational therapists. This paper will briefly describe the current issues related to manpower, recruitment and level II fieldwork education. It will then discuss the development, utilization and impact of one educational program designed to increase student interest in mental health by providing an opportunity for additional contact with senior clinicians during the level II fieldwork experience. In conclusion, this paper will give suggestions for future strategies that may lead to improved level II educational experiences as well as increased student interest in mental health as a career choice.

LITERATURE REVIEW

Manpower Trends

Today, occupational therapy manpower is limited while employment opportunities are increasing (American Occupational Therapy Association, 1985, 1987). Between 1966 and 1978 the occupational therapy workforce grew 170 percent. Since 1978, the annual rate of growth has declined (American Occupational Therapy Association, 1985, 1987; Berman, 1988; Fine, 1986, 1987; Gibson, 1986). Shortages in occupational therapy personnel are currently being reported by the National Task Force on Gerontology and Geriatric Care and the American Society of Allied Health Professionals (*OT*

Week, 1988). New job openings for allied health personnel are expected to grow at a rate far exceeding the overall average job growth in the U.S. economy by the year 2000 (*OT Week*, 1988). In 1986, according to the Member Data Survey, only 8.5 percent of occupational therapists identified themselves as mental health practitioners (American Occupational Therapy Association, 1987; Berman, 1988). This is particularly disturbing given the fact that approximately 50 years ago most occupational therapists worked in mental health (Gibson, 1986).

There are several possible explanations for the current shortage in occupational therapy personnel. Since 1977, the number of graduates from professional programs has not increased (American Occupational Therapy Association, 1985). Factors which have contributed to the decline in enrollment in professional programs include smaller numbers of college age students, escalating tuition costs and cut-backs in federal support for higher education (American Occupational Therapy Association, Winter, 1988; *OT Week*, March 17, 1988). As emphasis is placed on the recruitment of non-traditional students such as minorities, older students, individuals seeking a career change, persons with physical disabilities and men, schools still have yet to face the challenge of adjusting academic programs to meet these students' needs (*O.T. Week*, 1988; American Occupational Therapy Association, 1985). In addition, the occupational therapy manpower pool fluctuates due to a large percentage of its labor force taking time out from professional pursuits to raise a family. Currently, the profession includes only a small percentage of men and therapists with master's degrees, both of whom show a greater tendency to stay in the work force full-time (American Occupational Therapy Association, 1985). Finally, there still seems to be limited public awareness of occupational therapy as a viable career choice (*OT News*, March, 1988; Bonder, 1988).

Recruitment

General Recruitment Issues

At present, the issue of recruiting students into occupational therapy has held high visibility at both national and statewide levels. Five pilot tests of recruitment strategies have been described recently, reflecting a cooperative effort between AOTA, state associations, educational institutions and businesses. These pilot programs include: providing nationwide information to chairmen of biology and psychology departments about career opportunities; recruiting black students through specially designed recruitment brochures and radio announcements; and two statewide efforts to increase general public information about occupational therapy (*OT News*, March, 1988).

Several other recruitment strategies have been encouraged in the professional literature. One strategy calls for developing and advertising creative educational programs that will attract non-traditional students. Another strategy is to provide prospective students more chances to view occupational therapy in action as well as to have therapists speak at high school and college career days. Publishing information about the effectiveness of occupational therapy across professional journals and establishing more scholarships for student training may support recruitment efforts. Creating and advertising job benefit packages that would include flexible schedules, better salaries, more career laddering and on-site child care will help recruit non-traditional students and retain qualified professionals. (American Occupational Therapy Association, Winter, 1988; Berman, 1988; Bonder, 1988; *OT Week*, 1988; *OT Week*, 1988; Strickland, 1987). It has also been suggested that promotional activities target minorities, second career seekers, underemployed persons in related fields and baccalaureate degree graduates in related fields (American Occupational Therapy Association, 1985).

Recruitment into Mental Health Practice

Occupational therapists in mental health must look to the above recruitment strategies to encourage new or second career students to enter the field. Mental health practitioners must ensure that all general professional recruitment activities include appropriate examples of the variety of career opportunities available to therapists working in mental health.

Mental health practitioners face a challenge to stimulate and maintain students' interest in this area as the students proceed through their academic and clinical fieldwork experiences. Christie,

Joyce and Moeller (1985 a) found that out of 131 registered occupational therapists, 62% of the respondents identified the level II fieldwork experience as the stage having the greatest impact on their choice of a career specialty. The quality of the supervisory relationship was most frequently mentioned in this study as critical to a good fieldwork experience. Important components to this relationship were described as: (1) the supervisor being a good role model; (2) the supervisor being competent and confident in his/her clinical role; (3) the supervisor having enthusiasm for taking on the supervisory role; (4) the supervisor possessing teaching skills required to provide an individualized learning experience; and (5) the supervisor having good communication skills including the ability to give timely and constructive feedback. Christie, Joyce and Moeller (1985b) state,

> In summary, a consistent picture emerges as to what constitutes an effective and an ineffective supervisor. The effective supervisor fulfills basic supervisory responsibilities with strong interpersonal skills and with attitudes of supportiveness, interest, flexibility, and enthusiasm. The ineffective supervisor lacks essential interpersonal and organizational skills and, furthermore, displays negative personal attitudes such as unsupportiveness, rigidity, lack of enthusiasm, and insensitivity toward others. (pg. 677)

Wittman, Swinehart, St. Michel and Cahill (1988) noted that one of the two most important aspects of a high quality psychosocial fieldwork placement was the supervision provided. These authors indicated an increase in the number of students interested in mental health after the completion of the level II fieldwork placement.

Despite this powerful data, both clinical fieldwork supervisors and academic fieldwork coordinators experience difficulty accommodating students in quality level II psychosocial fieldwork experiences (Cohn & Frum, 1988; Frum, 1986). Fieldwork placements are often adversely affected by understaffed departments, limited availability of senior clinicians to provide supervision, limited time to perform supervision, few incentives for therapists to become supervisors and difficulty justifying educational programs in light of unmet service needs and shrinking resources. Student supervisors often begin supervising early in their careers, without the benefit of any formal training or ongoing supervision specific to their development as a student supervisor (Bonder, 1988; Christie et al., 1985b; Cohn & Frum, 1988). In Christie et al.'s study (1985b), 21% of the 188 student supervisors had less than the full year of clinical experience required by the "Guide to Fieldwork Education" (AOTA, 1984). In a national survey conducted by AOTA regional fieldwork consultants (Frum, 1986), the majority of fieldwork supervisors who responded had only one year of experience. Although it appears that the fieldwork experience is valued as an essential part of the profession's educational process, little attention has been directed to helping therapists learn how to be effective supervisors (Cohn & Frum, 1988; Crist, 1986), or to maintaining standards of education set by AOTA. "Fieldwork educators are expected to solidify the occupational therapy students' professional training, yet their primary role is patient care. Their expertise is in various clinical areas and skills rather than in supervision theory and practice" (Cohn & Frum, 1988, p. 325). Consequently, in order to develop and maintain students' interest in psychosocial occupational therapy as a career choice, it appears that particular attention must be paid to improving the supervisory process during the level II fieldwork experience.

Development of an Educational Seminar
for Level II Students

A variety of approaches are needed to help improve the level II fieldwork experience for both supervisors and supervisees. One strategy in current use revolves around the development of continuing education materials for beginning therapists, such as the material developed by Frum and Opacich (1987), and by Crist (1986). Educational institutions and state associations are providing more opportunities for therapists to participate in continuing education workshops and courses related to supervision.

Despite heightened awareness of the need to improve the educational preparation of student supervisors, we are still faced with the acute dilemma of how to enhance the educational experience of level II students who are currently completing their fieldwork placements in mental health. One approach to this problem is supplementation of the supervisory relationship by increasing the student's exposure to additional senior clinicians. This paper will review the development, utilization and impact of one educational program offered by a clinical setting to all level II fieldwork students in a metropolitan area. The educational program was designed to enrich the psychiatric level II experience by; (1) introducing students to a number of senior professionals working in a cross-section of mental health practice, (2) providing students information about the variety of roles and functions occupational therapists can assume in mental health, (3) offering examples of how senior professionals have developed their careers in mental health, and (4) providing a forum for senior clinicians to respond to student's questions and concerns about occupational therapy in mental health. It was hypothesized that this type of educational experience would be one efficient way to enhance the psychiatric level II experience and encourage students to consider seriously a career in mental health.

THE EDUCATIONAL PROGRAM

The program was available to all interested level II fieldwork students. Invitations were issued in two ways. One set of invitations was mailed to occupational therapy schools and a second set of invitations was sent to level II fieldwork settings. In this way, the program coordinators hoped to reach all eligible students. This approach depended on the cooperation of university faculty and fieldwork supervisors, all of whom were extremely enthusiastic and helpful. Students were readily released from placements to attend this seminar.

Students were invited, at no fee, to spend the day with identified experts in psychosocial occupational therapy. The program consisted of three "Keynote" addresses and two sessions of small group presentations. The large group "Keynote" addresses were designed to convene the participants and introduce them to three generations of distinguished professionals. (The content of these presentations is contained in this special issue.) After completing pre-program questionnaires, students heard two of the three major presentations. Small group presentations occurred during the middle portion of the day. Three presentations ran simultanously for the first hour, and three different presentations ran simultaneously for the second hour. Small group presentors were selected based on their expertise in "sub-specialties" of psychosocial occupational therapy. After the two small group sessions, the third major presentation culminated the day. At the conclusion of the seminar, students were asked to complete a final program questionnaire.

STUDENT PARTICIPANTS

Information about the student group was gleaned from the pre-program questionnaire. Fifty-five students from twelve different schools of occupational therapy were present. The majority were from schools in the New York City area, but some came from as far north as Boston, Massachusetts and as far south as Baltimore, Maryland. Most students were in the third month of their fieldwork placement in mental health; three were in adult physical disabilities settings; one student was in a pediatric setting; and one was completing a placement in gerontology.

Readiness for entry-level positions was quite variable, as only nine were completing fieldwork by the fall of 1988 and only twenty-five were scheduled to complete fieldwork by December, 1989. Thus, only slightly more than half the group was within weeks or months of committing to a speciality choice. The remaining twenty-one students were in their first fieldwork placements and would be in a variety of clinical and educational settings before making an initial career decision.

Student ages ranged from twenty to over fifty years of age. Thirty-three of these students (60%) were between twenty and twenty-five years old. More than half the group (thirty) were in undergraduate programs. Only two of the participants were male. Finally, twenty-six of the students (47%) reported some volunteer or salaried work experience in occupational therapy or a related field prior to beginning their academic studies.

Regarding the issue of specialty selection, students reported the following data: Of the twenty-nine students reporting having already made a specialty selection (53% of the total group), seven had definitely chosen mental health and seven more reported mental health as one of their considerations. The remaining twenty-six students had not yet made a specialty choice.

In relation to role modeling and mentorship, data revealed some interesting trends. Forty students (73%) had contact with occupational therapists before entering occupational therapy school. Only 4 students reported that this early contact with psychiatric occupational therapists had had an impact on current views of specialty choice.

While in their fieldwork settings, students reported that supervisors with five to fifteen years experience provided the best role models. In addition, 21% of the group reported that they felt their supervisor was not a good role model. These respondents described their supervisors as unaware of current assessments or theory, "burned out," insecure in their role, unavailable to the students, disorganized, or poorly skilled clinicians. During fieldwork placements, 76% of the students reported finding excellent role models in therapists other than their immediate supervisors. Many students also reported having found good role models prior to their fieldwork experience. A vast majority of these role models came from academic settings.

As other background information, students were asked to identify three qualities that they would look for in a professional role model. These qualities are listed in descending order of frequency of identification:

1. Strong fund of professional knowledge, extensive work experience and effective clinical reasoning skills (46 students);
2. Confidence in ability to define and assert role as an occupational therapist when working with other team members. (28 students);
3. Combines professional attitude with a warm and energetic personality (24 students);
4. Skilled clinician who combines creative treatment plans with empathy and caring (23 students);
5. Dedicated to the profession, a hard worker and committed to continued learning (17 students);

6. Good communication and supervisory skills (15 students);
7. Well organized (9 students);
8. Good leadership skills (4 students).

Finally, all 55 students were asked to identify one question they would like to have answered about occupational therapy in mental health. The purpose of this exercise was to engage students in thinking about what they wanted to know about psychosocial occupational therapy. It also provided some background information to the authors about questions students were grappling with at this stage of their professional development. Of this group, 58% of the students were able to clearly formulate at least one question that they wanted the senior clinicians to answer during the course of the seminar. Students questions were the following in order of frequency;

- What are the career opportunities in mental health both now and in the future?
- What is the role of a psychiatric occupational therapist working with different patient populations?
- How are occupational therapists different from other professionals in a psychiatric setting?
- How difficult is it to open a private practice in psychiatry?
- How do you explain psychiatric occupational therapy to people outside the profession?
- How do you motivate the uninterested patient?
- What is the pay scale in mental health? Is the pay scale lower then in other specialties?
- If you do not have a lot of experience with formal occupational therapy assessments, can you get this training in your first job?
- How effective is psychiatric occupational therapy?
- Why is there such a strong delineation between occupational therapy in psychiatry and physical dysfunction?
- Should supervisory training be included in occupational therapy curriculum, as entry level therapists are often expected to provide supervision?
- How much respect does the psychiatric occupational therapist get as part of the treatment team?

PROGRAM RESULTS

At the end of the seminar 43 of the original 55 students, 80%, completed a final program questionnaire. Of this group,14 participants (32%) reported that they received some answers to their original questions and 12 (28%) stated they received no answer. The other 17 students (40%) did not respond or indicated they had not posed an original question. Participants' written comments about what they learned included the following: (1) Acquired more information about occupational therapy treatment with different psychiatric populations; (2) Increased their awareness of important psychosocial issues that can be applied to their work in physical disabilities; (3) Discovered that salaries in psychiatry were better than anticipated; (4) Learned about the role of occupational therapy in relation to other psychiatric disciplines; (5) Increased knowledge about current trends in psychiatric occupational therapy; (6) Increased their awareness of the diversity of long term career opportunities in mental health; (7) Felt more aware of the important role occupational therapy can play in mental health; (8) Gained a greater awareness of the importance of good supervision to the beginning therapist; and (9) Increased their knowledge of the interpersonal and leadership skills required to become a good therapist.

Other feedback from students included the following information. A majority of the respondents (90%) felt that the educational seminar reinforced or increased their knowledge of the role of the occupational therapist in mental health. In addition, 35% of the respondents reported that the seminar was effective in influencing their future specialty selection. All of the respondent found an average of 3 role models from the group of senior clinicians. Students noted that the top three qualities that made the presenters most appealing were their fund of knowledge, their style of presentation and their interpersonal skills. When asked which type of group format they preferred, 40% of the students preferred the small groups, 30% preferred the large groups and 30% liked the combination of both types of group presentations. When students were asked if the seminar affected their specialty choice within the field of occupational therapy, eleven (25%) stated that it either prompted or solidified their decision to work in psychiatry. Thirteen (30%) reported they were still undecided, with half of this group commenting that their interest in psychiatry had increased. Nineteen (44%) reported no change in their decision to pursue a specialty outside of psychiatry, and five of these indicated that the program had increased their awareness of the importance of psychosocial issues in physical rehabilitation.

At the completion of the seminar, 86% of the students completing the questionnaire reported being satisfied to very satisfied with the content of the day long educational seminar. The three most frequent comments included: (1) It was good to hear from seniors in the field who are pleased with their work and can provide "inspiration" to others; (2) The seminar was well organized and informative; and finally, (3) There was a good variety of speakers. Suggestions given by students for future educational experiences of this nature included: (1) providing more breaks between presentations; (2) providing more time in both large and small groups for senior clinicians to answer questions and have informal discussions; and (3) providing more chances for students to attend small groups. Finally, a large percentage of the students indicated that this type of educational seminar should be repeated in the future.

The presentors were also asked to complete a post-seminar questionnaire. In this questionnaire all of the presentors indicated that they both enjoyed participating in the seminar and felt it was well organized. When asked for feedback, they agreed with the students that there was not enough time for informal discussion in both the large and small groups. They also suggested that more structured breaks might have made the day more palatable for all.

PROGRAM EXPENSES

Prior to initiating such a recruitment program, institutions, either academic or clinical, must consider costs. An estimate of expenses should include both direct and indirect costs. Indirect costs should include the value of the presentors' donated time as well as the value of staff hours taken away from regular administrative and clinical duties at the sponsoring institution. Future financial recommendations for delivering such a program are: (1) Charging students a small registration fee; (2) Seeking financial support from local academic or fieldwork sites; (3) Exploring the possibility of financial support from local mental health special interest groups; and (4) Providing an honorarium for the presentors. In addition, it is important to pursue careful tracking of the outcome of such a program in relation to it's costs. In this day of shrinking resources, cost effective programs are of utmost importance.

DISCUSSION

Although the information reported in this article is only from one small group of level II fieldwork students who are from a similar geographical area, several interesting themes emerge that may merit consideration by the profession's leaders, educators and clinical supervisors. First, though many students have contact with occupational therapists prior to beginning their academic studies, few of these therapists work in psychiatry. In addition, it appears that there are an increasing number of older students pursuing a masters degree in occupational therapy but still a very limited number of males. In relation to role models, it appears that students have multiple role models available to them via school and fieldwork experiences. It is unclear from the information that was collected, however, how many of these role models worked in the area of psychiatric occupational therapy. In addition, it is unknown how much access students have to identified role models when they need information and/or help in making future career decisions.

In relation to supervision, it is surprising to note that unlike information in the literature (Christie et al., 1985b; Frum, 1986), many of the students did have supervisors with several years of clinical experience. It seems that the least successful supervisory experiences occurred with clinicians who had less than two years of experience or with supervisors who were described by students as being "burned out." It is noteable that this group of students felt the best supervision was provided by clinicians with 5 to 15 years of experience. Qualities that identified good supervisors and good role models are similar to those cited in the literature. Some of the most important positive supervisory/role model traits appear to be those that require several years of clinical work to acquire. These traits include fund of knowledge, professional confidence, clinical expertise and sense of professional commitment. Other important traits are related to the supervisor's communication and teaching skills which supervisors frequently develop without the support of any formal training.

It is disturbing to note that although 90% of the program participants were in their third month of their psychiatric fieldwork, many reported still not understanding the role of an occupational therapist in a psychiatric setting. This lack of understanding could be related to the students never being taught this information or the students needing to have this information repeated in order to confirm or integrate knowledge being learned (Frum & Opacich, 1987; Schwartz, 1984). It might also be due to the general anxiety that students feel as they anticipate having to move into professional roles. Finally, students may be reflecting the role confusion they have experienced from their supervisors.

Many participants did not feel they had adequate information about the variety of career opportunities that are available in psychiatric occupational therapy. Among students who had clearly chosen a career in a non-psychiatric specialty, many noted that the seminar had made them more sensitive to the psychosocial issues of the non-psychiatric patients with whom they were working.

Although there is no data currently available about how many of the students who participated in this program actually chose to work in psychiatric occupational therapy, it appears that the program helped to maintain and/or stimulate several participants' interest. Several students who were questioning their original interest in psychiatry due to unsatisfactory supervisory experiences, reported that the program helped rekindle their original interest. Providing a continuing education program addressed important learning needs for the majority of the program participants at a pivotal juncture in their professional training.

RECOMMENDATIONS

Psychiatric occupational therapists must be involved in recruitment efforts that bring eligible students with a general interest in psychiatry to the field of occupational therapy. Once recruited, it appears that the level II fieldwork experience may be the critical time period to maintain or generate interest in mental health as a career specialty choice. To insure that this "critical period" is a high quality training experience, the profession must make an increased commitment to the training of its fieldwork supervisors. Several suggestions are found in the literature on how to improve fieldwork education (Cohn & Frum, 1988; Christie et al., 1985b; Crist, 1986; Still, 1982). These proposals and the suggestions of the authors are summarized as follows:

1. Encourage greater adherance to AOTA guidelines for fieldwork supervision.
2. Fieldwork sites should consider assigning students to senior therapists whenever possible. This will allow junior therapists to increase their clinical fund of knowledge, to gain experience in applying theory to clinical situations, and to develop a sense of self-confidence as a clinician prior to assuming supervisory responsibilities.
3. Require that all occupational therapists attend a standardized supervisory training program in order to earn the credentials necessary to become a student supervisor. This will provide potential supervisors with information on supervisory theory, learning theory, communication skills and student evaluation. It will also increase supervisors' awareness of the important role they play in both student training and student career specialty choice. This continuing education program could be developed nationally through AOTA and implemented through state associations.
4. Initiate a national supervisory special interest group available to both student and staff supervisors.
5. Increase the number of self-study tools available to new supervisors.
6. Increase national and local support for level II fieldwork educational seminars such as the one described in this paper.
7. Increase the association between senior clinicians and academic programs by inviting more clinicians to participate in the classroom.
8. Require that academic programs include an introductory

course on the utilization of professional supervision. This would help students anticipate the fieldwork learning process, discuss typical ways that anxiety can affect learning and raise student consciousness about their roles and responsibilities within the context of the supervisory experience.

9. Start an "Educational Column" in *O.T. Week* addressing issues relevant to students and supervisors.

In conclusion, it appears that some of the above recommendations may help to improve the level II fieldwork experience in psychiatry and therefore influence students career choice. Certainly many of the above suggestions would also benefit the entire profession, since student supervisors across all specialty areas face the same lack of formal training related to supervision.

CONCLUSION

This article has provided information on the current manpower trends and recruitment issues facing occupational therapists today. It highlighted several recruitment strategies that are currently being applied by the profession to increase the number of students entering academic programs in occupational therapy. Given the nationwide attention being paid to attracting students to the profession, the authors decided it was important to focus on the issue of how to sustain or to initiate students' interest in psychiatric occupational therapy once they were committed to the profession. Literature indicated that the level II fieldwork supervisory experience appeared to be a critical factor in a student's career specialty choice. Therefore a day long educational seminar was developed to enrich this fieldwork experience by providing students with the opportunity to have contact with three generations of senior occupational therapists. Results indicate that the seminar was a success in several ways. It increased a majority of the participants' knowledge about psychiatric occupational therapy. The seminar also helped confirm and stimulate some students' interest in psychiatric occupational therapy as a possible career choice. Information gleaned from the student group provided interesting feedback about student backgrounds, student perceptions of good role models and supervisors, and student's questions about psychiatric occupational therapy. Information gathered from current literature as well as feedback from program participants pointed to several of the recommendations made to improve the level II psychiatric fieldwork experience. It is hoped that improving the quality of these experiences will increase career interest in psychiatric occupational therapy. Further research studies are needed to better understand the process of students' career specialty selection.

REFERENCES

American Occupational Therapy Association (1984). *Guide to Fieldwork Education* (1986 ed.). Baltimore, MD: Commission on Education of the American Occupational Therapy Association.

American Occupational Therapy Association (1985). *Occupational therapy manpower: A plan for progress*. Rockville, MD: Author.

American Occupational Therapy Association (1987, September). Member data survey. Rockville, MD: Author.

Berman, C. B. (1988). Recruitment and retention: Approaches that work. In, *Proceedings of the Fifth Annual Preconference to the American Psychiatric Association's 40th Institute on Hospital & Community Psychiatry* (pp. 47-62). Rockville, MD: American Occupational Therapy Association, Inc.

Bonder, B. (1988, March). Mental health SIS annual meeting addresses professional issues. *Mental Health Special Interest Section Newsletter*, pp. 3-4.

Cohn, E. S. & Frum, D.C. (1988). Fieldwork supervision: More education is warranted. *American Journal of Occupational Therapy*, *42*, 325-327.

Christie, B. A., Joyce, P. C., & Mueller, P. L. (1985a). Fieldwork experience, part 1: Impact on practice preference. *American Journal of Occupational Therapy*, *39*, 671-674.

Christie, B. A., Joyce, P. C., & Mueller, P. L. (1985b). Fieldwork experience, part II: The supervisor's dilemma. *American Journal of Occupational Therapy*, *39*, 675-681.

Creative approaches urged for expanding labor pool of allied health professionals. (1988, July 28). *OT Week*, pp. 1, 31.

Crist, P. A. H. (1986). *Contemporary issues in clinical education*. New Jersey: Slack.

Critical OT shortage predicted: Allied health society reports growing problem. (1988, March 17). *OT Week*, p. 2.

Despite gloomy shortage projections opportunity exists for recruiting OTs. (1988, October 13). *OT Week*, pp. 1, 30.

Discover OT! (1988, Winter). *OT Education Bulletin*, p. 12.

Fine, S. B. (1986). Trends in mental health. In S. C. Robertson (Ed.) *Mental*

Health SCOPE (pp. 19-32). Rockville, MD: The American Occupational Therapy Association.

Fine, S.B. (1987). Looking ahead: Opportunities for occupational therapy in the next decade. *Occupational Therapy in Mental Health*, *7* 3-12.

Frum, D. C. (1986, July). Study shows fieldwork to be a high priority among occupational therapy educators. *OT News*. p. 7.

Frum, D. C. & Opacich, K. J. (1987). *Supervision: Development of therapeutic competence*. Rockville, MD: American Occupational Therapy Association.

Gibson, D. (1986). Staffing in mental health. In S. C. Robertson (Ed.) *Mental Health SCOPE* (pp. 33-40). Rockville, MD: The American Occupational Therapy Association.

Page, M. S., (1987, September). Factors that influence students' choice of mental health as a career. *Mental Health Special Interest Section Newsletter*, pp. 1-3.

Recruitment strategies: Model programs developed. (1988, March). *Occupational Therapy News*, p.5.

Schwartz, K. B. (1984). An approach to supervision of students on fieldwork. *American Journal of Occupational Therapy*, *38*, 393-397.

Still, J. R. (1982). Mini-councils: A solution to fieldwork supervision. *American Journal of Occupational Therapy*, *36*, 328-332.

Wittman, P., Swinehart, S., St. Michel, G., & Cahill, R. (1988). *Variables affecting specialty choice in occupational therapy practice*. Unpublished research study. (Available from the American Occupational Therapy Foundation.)

A Mid-Career Perspective
of Mental Health Practice

Mark S. Rosenfeld, PhD, OTR

SUMMARY. The mental health practice area in occupational therapy has contracted during the 1980s. The practice area has been stongly affected by changing social values, reimbursement requirements and demographic trends. This paper offers a perspective on the realities, challenges and benefits of a career in mental health occupational therapy. The paper may be used by educators and supervisors in discussing the psychosocial dysfunction practice area with students.

INTRODUCTION

Important challenges face the psychosocial dysfunction practice area. While mental health once comprised 20% of occupational therapy practice, in recent years the numbers of students entering psychiatric occupational therapy have decreased markedly (Bonder, 1987). Occupational therapists working in community mental health centers decreased by 50% between 1977 and 1982. During this same period, mental health practice has moved to the community, due to deinstitutionalization and cost containment efforts (AOTA Commission on Manpower, 1985). Despite this shift, the American Occupational Therapy Association manpower study found that most occupational therapists in mental health continue to work in inpatient settings. Moreover, only 36% are directly reim-

Mark S. Rosenfeld is Assistant Professor, Tufts University, Boston School of Occupational Therapy, Medford, MA 02155.

In August 1988, the Therapeutic Activities Department of the Payne-Whitney Clinic, New York Hospital, sponsored a conference for affiliating students. The following paper is adopted from the author's speech.

bursed for services. Some therapists report frustration with the diminishing length of inpatient care, since traditional treatment approaches require graded learning over time (Jackson, 1984).

Several authors have suggested adaptations in role definitions, evaluation, treatment, and documentation methods required for occupational therapists to function successfully in the context of shortened inpatient stays (Bradlee, 1984; Jackson, 1984; Kaplan, 1984; Short, 1984). Ethridge (1987) advocates a shift of services to the community. He states that therapists must be capable of functioning as generalist case-managers, consultants and private practitioners. Furthermore, they must be resourceful, creative and independent in diverse environments which often lack the secure structure of traditional clinical settings.

Flexible and well trained new practitioners will be required to meet such a challenge. A study of 58 occupational therapy students at Ohio State University, however, found many to be negatively disposed toward mental health (Page, 1987). Several contributing factors were identified, including the population, the content of practice and the practice environment. Some students were frightened of encountering violent, unpredictable patients. Others felt that positive treatment outcomes were uncertain in mental health. They also considered the practice environment to be unpleasant. With respect to these issues, Page found that negative impressions reflected little direct experience, or were based only upon early visits to state hospitals. Students' concern about practice content consisted of a dislike for the abstract, problem-solving process required in mental health. Page suggested that these students were cognitively and developmentally more comfortable with concrete solutions to problems which could be learned and applied with repeated success.

Despite the negatives, there are positive elements shaping the future of psychosocial dysfunction as well. Occupational therapists have begun to generate research to document the value of our services in mental health. The field of psychiatry, which strongly influences the establishment, design and staffing of mental health programs, has begun to adopt a psychosocial rehabilitation model the treatment of long-term patients (Fine, 1988). There are many people in the community in need of such rehabilitation. Public concern and legislative support for programs to help chronically disabled and homeless individuals is on the increase. The above factors represent opportunities for occupational therapy. To take advantage of these opportunities, however, the mental health practice area will need creative, independent practitioners prepared to define and justify their services. Therapists must be ready to work in the community itself, rather than in traditional, secure institutional settings (Jackson, 1984). Home-care and school system therapists can provide helpful models, since they have already made this transition with notable success.

If the trend among occupational therapy students away from mental health persists, and if practitioners remain in inpatient environments, opportunities will be lost. With these issues in mind, I will review my career as an occupational therapist in mental health in an effort to encourage students toward this area of practice.

THE IMPACT OF CHANGING SOCIAL FORCES

I began Columbia University's occupational therapy program in 1971. It was easy to choose mental health practice in those days. The values and social climate prevalent were quite different than those which bear on students' career decisions today.

In 1971, the civil rights and anti-war movements contributed to a spirit of growth and transformation of self and society. Johnson's "Great Society" had created many social programs, and a new respect for helping roles and professions, although salaries remained rather low. Ethnic, religious and social class diversity was valued as an enriching characteristic of our society. Over the last decade, however, we have returned to the values of "competitive individualism" (Gordon, 1988). The disadvantaged are now expected to pull themselves up by their bootstraps. Consistent with these ideas, argues Gordon, helping roles and helping professions are devalued. During this period, women have made great progress in the world of work. With improved career options, however, many are abandoning helping roles and occupations in favor of more lucrative professions.

In the present milieu, personal income has become increasingly important. In 1971, many students were financially supported by scholarships and low-cost loans. Access to such support has significantly diminished. Students have struggled to afford professional education, and by necessity, have become extremely pragmatic in planning their careers.

An occupational therapist can make a reasonable living these days. It seems doubtful that students' choice of a practice area will leave them either wealthy or impoverished. But large educational debts may make slight salary differentials seem highly significant to those choosing a first job. In as far as salaries in mental health lag in certain areas, student choices may be affected.

The emphasis on financial issues has influenced many occupational therapists to take an entrepreneurial approach to their work. Private contracting has become a popular option, since therapists are currently in a strong marketplace position due to severe personnel shortages. Since there are few occupational therapists to provide adequate role modeling in private mental health practice, ambitious students may be discouraged from pursuing a specialty in this area.

Sweeping changes have occurred in our field in response to the shifting social climate described above. The health care system is driven by the profit motive and by cost containment, competing forces that are difficult to reconcile. The burgeoning cost of health care has taught us that thrift and accountability are extremely important. However, third party payers contain costs by stringently limiting services to consumers (Richards, 1984). Meanwhile, profits made by private hospitals, drug and equipment companies and by some health professionals, continue to rise. In discussing the growing emphasis on cost-benefit analysis, Brodie and Banner warn, "Realistic thinking does not assume that we can solve our health care crisis by a strict reliance on numbers; you cannot crunch numbers in this field without crunching lives" (1988, p.64).

I have seen many patients discharged prematurely and without adequate provision for aftercare, under pressure from insurance companies. Even in these cases, some hospitals made money by piling up bills for testing and specialized services of questionable necessity. Such strategies will lead to even more stringent efforts to limit services, and increase the burden of health care costs on consumers and society at large.

RISKS FOR OCCUPATIONAL THERAPY AND MENTAL HEALTH

Occupational therapists, rarely control the policy decisions that restrict patient care. Nor is there reason to suggest that therapists make profits based upon unethical practices. Nonetheless, our field is profoundly influenced by its participation in service systems, and by its efforts to adapt to prevailing conditions.

Occupational therapy, striving to make its way in a competitive universe, must be careful not to be lured far from its organizing beliefs. As treatment is defined by billing requirements, therapists are at risk for spending more time documenting and less time treating. Reductionistic methods are increasingly employed, since they lend themselves to measurable and predictable outcomes, which are reimbursable. Rogers (1982, p. 35) indicates that our philosophy differs from the medical emphasis on health, in that it "involves the presence as opposed to the absence of a quality, it implies activity rather than passivity, it encompasses psychological, social and environmental dimensions as well as biological; and it uses an optimum versus a minimum standard."

Will the quality of life of a whole person be gradually abandoned as a treatment focus? People, after all, possess free will, and are therefore, less predictable than are neurons, hand functions, or even depressive symptoms. Given the current milieu, the latter are far more suitable foci for billable treatment plans. Principled therapists must often justify their efforts to understand the life contexts within which their patients function, and to appreciate their aspirations and fears.

During this time of personnel shortage, many occupational therapists have developed private consulting and contracting firms. They often serve institutions which need the OTR initials to meet regulatory agency requirements, but which have neither the funding nor the will to provide adequate occupational therapy services to meet their patients' needs.

Mental health occupational therapy has been more negatively affected by these trends than has any other practice area. It has always been strongly committed to a holistic philosophy, assessing and mobilizing the unique potentials of the individual or group. Interventions are shaped by the characteristics of the patient and his or her functional environment. Perhaps these precepts have made mental health less precise and therefore, less reimbursable, less adaptable to current circumstances than are other areas of occupational therapy practice. Adaptation, however, is not always entirely positive. What seems functional in the current context, may erode the philosophical base of the profession, and exact entrepreneurial benefit at the expense of the patients we serve.

I believe that we must address the current challenge by:

1. Developing and promoting innovative, community-based programs for populations in need;
2. Working actively with other disciplines and with clients to design and market these programs to funding sources;
3. Demonstrating the effectiveness of our services by routine evaluation of concrete program accomplishments;
4. Working with patients and families against legislation, social attitudes and institutional policies that dehumanize treatment, reduce standards of care and denegrate quality of life considerations;
5. Scrutinize our own practices so as to identify and modify circumstances that promote high pay and institutional profits in return for minimal service.

Our contribution and commitment to patient care justifies the existence of our profession. While our services have always been economically undervalued, we must not accept popular practices that compromise our commitment to patients.

Despite recent setbacks, I have always felt that psychiatric occupational therapy is intrinsically strong. It makes important and unique contributions to patients' lives. Practitioners in this area are generally insightful, effective people who have accomplished a great deal in collaboration with patients. In the section which follows, the strengths of mental health occupational therapy practice will be illustrated, and each of the previously identified areas of student concern will be addressed.

POPULATION

Experience does not corroborate the concerns of the Ohio State students. Although some psychiatric patients may temporarily lose control, I have not found many patients to be threatening or violent. The work has been upsetting and taxing at times. And there are some good reasons for students to feel frightened. Most fears encountered in supervision sessions with students, however, involve the potential for failure and narcissistic injury rather than physical assault. These fears seem to come with the territory. In mental health practice, there is often intensive interaction between patients and staff. Staff may feel vulnerable and exposed, unable to gain the protection of a formal role or a standard technique. Students and therapists must learn to cope with the following fears:

- I may be so different from patients that I cannot understand or help them;
- I may be like the patients in some respects, and this realization frightens me;
- I may hate some patients, and therefore, fail as a therapist;
- I may be so emotionally affected by patients that I "catch" their feelings;
- I may identify with patients, confront my own problems, and feel overwhelmed;
- My imperfections as a person (therapist) may cause me to provoke or injure patients;
- My imperfections will be evident to patients (and staff) and I will be rejected;
- Patients' problems may be too overwhelming for me to solve;
- I may not be authoritative in setting limits, and be challenged by patients;
- I may be effective in setting limits, but be hated by patients as a result;

—I may feel guilty about the relative advantages and successes I've had in life;

—Patients may be cruel and out of control of their anger, and assault me.

These fears are normal, understandable and surmountable when responsibilities are graded and effective supervision is offered. It takes time to get used to a culture in which it is considered normal to hear the most intimate life details and feelings of relative strangers.

Sooner or later, an occupational therapist in mental health will encounter patients with family problems and divorce, job and economic failures, physical or sexual abuse, psychosis, out of control alcohol and drug use, and suicidal depression. I've worked with welfare mothers, investment bankers, refugees, angry teenagers, and older adults in decline, people of every conceivable geographic and ethnic background. These enriching experiences have taught me a great deal about life, other people, and myself. I've gotten to know countless people I never would have met in my narrower social milieu. In the context of treatment, I've discovered these people to be unique and often quite different from my biased initial impressions. In many instances, hope and renewal have been forged through the occupational therapy experience.

AMBIGUITY OF PRACTICE

Students' concern that mental health practice offers no set answers or clearly predictable results is understandable. The complexity and ambiguity of psychiatric treatment, and developmental self-doubts, led me to feel inadequate as a therapist for some time after I graduated from Columbia University. Upon meeting a new patient, I would ask of myself as many questions as I asked the patient in an effort to grasp the person and situation at hand. Eventually, these anxious but appropriate questions led me to a good evaluation and a focused treatment process. From talking and doing, the crucible of experience, we can understand who patients are, the swirl of their personal life contexts, and how to help them realize the futures they desire.

Occupational therapists break seemingly insurmountable problems into manageable goals and tasks. A good therapeutic process is like alchemy that works. Ordinary actions, words and ideas become charged with meaning. Action, reflection and insight tumble over each other in stimulating and valuable ways. Every moment is one of functioning, of observation, and discovery.

> Because the simplest of life tasks (preparing a meal, using the telephone, or filing a letter) represents the complex integration of multiple factors, a systematic consideration of these components facilitates a fuller understanding of patterns of past, current and potential function. (Fine, 1983, p. 6)

Of course, much of therapy is just good hard work, not always spectacular. The value of the work to the patient depends upon the selection and performance of occupations that address salient functional and developmental concerns, and that provide clear avenues for observable growth. I refer to such occupations as nuclear tasks, since they are central to problem or crisis resolution (Rosenfeld, 1984).

In my experience, a treatment relationship is therapeutic if it enables the patient, in partnership, to identify and surmount obstacles to improved performance and/or satisfaction in daily occupations. Therapeutic interactions involve the following steps:

1. Address and examine functional history, current patterns and future goals;
2. Reframe problems in a functional skill context;
3. Value and investigate the unique potentials, perspectives and identity of the patient;
4. Move from reflecting to planning to doing in a measured and productive sequence;
5. Offer expert consultation about occupational options, sequences, and performance;
6. Stress the patient's responsibility for decisions and actions which affect the quality of his/her life;
7. Use reality awareness as a template against which to view the patient's decisions and actions;
8. Support growth through gradual skill development, facing

manageable risks, and accurately assessing productive efforts as well as end products;

9. Foster the patient's self-observing and problem-solving capacities so that occupational functioning will persist and improve beyond termination.

Occupational therapists certainly have strong "medicine" at their disposal. Years ago, Endicott and Spitzer, important contributors to the development of *DSM III.* conducted a longitudinal study of patients from New York State Psychiatric Institute. Although few patients surveyed remembered their doctor's name or their medications five years after discharge, it was reported to me that without being asked, many patients recalled an occupational therapist with whom they had worked, and a project they had completed. Mastery during a time of helplessness and confusion, can have a lasting impact. Skillful cuing and structuring by a therapist enables patients to mobilize and use capacities that are just emerging into a zone of proximal development, and which they may not yet be able to draw upon alone (Lyons, 1984). The following vignettes illustrate the growth that can occur in the context of occupational therapy practice in mental health.

CASE VIGNETTES

Jennifer

A suicidal 14 year old girl had been sexually abused and had drifted into a life of promiscuous sex and drug abuse. During her hospitalization, whatever activity we undertook, from softball to poetry writing, it was the first time for Jennifer. Her fund of occupational experience was incredibly sparse. After completing a wristband project near the end of her hospitalization, she said, "You know what all these activities mean for me? They mean I can finally be my age. I can do the things that other kids do now, and I'm not so bad at a lot of them either." Could anyone have said it better?

Alice

Alice was a schizophrenic woman in her fifties, who was admitted to the hospital non-psychotic, but severely depressed. She had gradually stopped functioning in her role as homemaker, and felt that her husband now hated her, since he was burdened with full-time work and the household chores as well. Family therapy proved unproductive for the couple, neither of whom were verbally oriented. An occupational therapy evaluation consisting of a baking task, showed that husband tended to take over, underestimate wife's abilities, and that she passively sat by while he baked. No communication occurred. No decision-making, support, feedback, or socializing took place between them. The therapist offered concrete feedback about these deficiencies and their impact. The couple gingerly began working together. The next session took place at the family's neighborhood supermarket. Husband drove. He jumped into the perceived void once again, picking up groceries and placing them in the cart, but the therapist intervened. Alice then selected foods while husband pushed the cart. They conferred about choices and prices. After checking and paying the bill together, the couple left the store smiling. Husband had his arm around Alice's shoulders. There was music in the air.

Sam

Sam was a young man struggling to recover from his first psychotic break. He had lost trust in his judgement and self-control. In woodworking, he faced the challenge of a circular saw. With real trepidation and with close support, Sam handled the rather intimidating tool with care and control. His sense of self began to shift in a positive direction on the hinge of that experience.

Emilio

Emilio was a man in his forties who had been a small time gangster before his divorce and trouble with his bosses precipitated a psychotic episode. After discharge, he lived in a single room occupancy hotel room which he hated. He felt degraded by the dirty, roach-infested environment. Nonetheless, Emilio came to day treatment in a suit and tie most days. These clothes were a symbol of his self-respect. But he could never save money for a better apartment, because of his cleaning bills. He did not know how to do laundry, and took all his clothes to the cleaners. A visit to his room revealed that there were no shelves or closet space for his clothing. Together, we did the laundry, and opened a savings account with the money he saved by avoiding the cleaners. We built a closet with shelves and a hanger rack in his room. And a little bit, we rebuilt hope for the future.

*   *   *

There are many more people, tasks, and stories. Therapists create their own vignettes, and their own excitement. There is excitement in the work. It is present in mental health practice, and it always has been, despite the apprehensions of Page's students.

PRACTICE ENVIRONMENT

My practice environments have been quite varied. I've worked in state, voluntary and private hospitals, and in private practice. I have run a day treatment program and an occupational therapy department in an acute-care hospital, taught in a number of educational programs, and recently worked at Red Cross with disaster victims. At 42, I honestly don't know where the future will lead. My professional activities have also been quite varied. After graduation, my opportunities quickly broadened to include advanced study, administration, teaching, consulting, research, writing and private practice. Excellent, diverse opportunities are still available for new therapists entering the profession.

One of the truly wonderful elements of mental health practice has involved working in the context of a therapeutic milieu, and in therapeutic communities. They are laboratories for learning. I often found these communities to be more tolerant, humane, open and effective than groups and organizations in the world at large. People have real influence and impact upon each other, even in acute care settings, in which community makeup is constantly shifting. As an occupational therapist, I have helped patients to solve problems, to take new roles and effective actions. Thereby they have gathered strength, courage and skills for life beyond treatment. The following are examples of milieu work.

Thirty-five inpatients had real trouble sharing a single washer and dryer. It was a mess. Clothing was always left in the machines, arguments occurred over turns at the dryer. I helped the group to plan and build shelves for the laundry room, sorting and storing clothes. We formulated and posted rules for using the machines, and a community job to monitor and clean the room was created. Minor functional efforts avoided major interpersonal tensions.

A large group of adolescents wanted only to do vandalism as a way of celebrating Halloween. Annoyed at being in a restrictive inpatient setting, they refused to plan a party. Using activity analysis skills, I devised a marshmallow war as a non-destructive vehicle for aggressive fun. The air rained marshmallows for five minutes, until everyone was tired. No one was hurt, because the marshmallows just bounced off, no matter how hard they were thrown. Everyone had a great time, and the adolescents were then able to join the adults for a good party.

Weekend planning has always been a challenge. In day treatment, patients often seemed anxious as the treatment week came to a close. We instituted a "Dear Day Center" activity at Friday's lunch, modeled after Dear Abby. Patients wrote problems, concerns and statements anonymously on 3 × 5 cards. The community read them aloud, and offered advice and empathy in return. Concrete plans to structure weekend time often emerged from this process, and the Friday transition always seemed easier thereafter. Concrete planning with activity configuration has always been extremely valuable for patients working toward discharge. As planned activities for life outside fill the schedule, anxiety abates.

In the course of community work, I have refined my values as a social being, and improved my skills in dealing with an incredible range of issues. I will always value this element of occupational therapy practice, even if third party payers do not.

Active experience with patients and a functional orientation enabled me to bring vital information to the interdisciplinary team process. Functional assessment has become even more important since discharge often follows so closely on the heels of admission. Team members are frequently uncertain about testing results indicating perceptual or neurological deficits, cognitive dysfunction, motor or learning disabilities. An occupational therapist can report from direct experience, how these problems impact on the patient's functioning. The full range of knowledge acquired in occupational therapy education, is certainly valuable in psychosocial dysfunction practice, given the diversity of problems encountered in treatment.

CONCLUSION

Many practice opportunities exist in the community. For example, the homeless are in great need of functional rehabilitation, and some therapists have already joined that effort. Forty percent of teenagers in a recent study were reported unable to accurately make change for a purchase or fill out a summer job application (Cetron, 1988). Certainly, additional occupational therapy services are needed in American communities. We will require both resourceful leaders and energetic new practitioners to succeed in offering these services. The philosophy, ethics, theories and methods of our field provide a strong springboard. But we therapists must spring and dive with exacting form and grace.

Working in psychosocial dysfunction has been terrific. If students are up to the risks and challenges, and if they can tolerate some early insecurity, then mental health can be right for them too. An East Indian poet once wrote,

> The faith waiting in the heart of a seed
> promises a miracle of life
> which it cannot prove at once.

—Tagore, 1928, p. 85

REFERENCES

American Occupational Therapy Association. (1985). *Occupational Therapy Manpower: A Plan For Progress*. Rockville, Md.

Bonder, B. (1987). Occupational therapy in mental health: crisis or opportunity? *American Journal of Occupational Therapy, 41*, 495-499.

Bradlee, L. (1984). The use of groups in short-term psychiatric settings. *Occupational Therapy in Mental Health,4*, 47-57.

Cetron, M. (1988, August). Teach our children well. *Omni*, p. 14.

Ethridge, D. (1987, March 26). Mental health issues shifting . . . need grows for independents. *O. T. Week*, pp. 4-5.

Fidler, G. & Fidler, J. (1978). Doing and becoming: purposeful action and self-actualization. *American Journal of Occupational Therapy*, *32*, 305-310.

Fine, S. (1983). Occupational therapy: the role of rehabilitation and purposeful activity in mental health practice. Rockville, Md.: American Occupational Therapy Association.

Gordon, S. (1988, July). The crisis in caring. *Boston Globe Magazine*, pp. 22-73.

Jackson, G. (1984). Short-term psychiatric treatment: how will occupational therapy adapt? *Occupational Therapy in Mental Health*, *4*, pp. 11-17.

Kaplan, K. (1984). Short-term assessment: the need and a response. *Occupational Therapy in Mental Health*, *4*, pp. 29-45.

Lyons, B. (1984). Defining a child's zone of proximal development: evaluation process for treatment planning. *American Journal of Occupational Therapy*, *38*, 446-451.

Page, M. (1987, September). Factors that influence students' choice of mental health as a career. *Mental Health Special Interest Section Newsletter*, pp. 1-3.

Richards, G. (1984). Technology costs and rationing issues. *Hospitals*, *58*, pp. 80-88.

Rogers, J. (1982). Order and disorder in medicine and occupational therapy. *American Journal of Occupational Therapy*, *36*, 29-35.

Rosenfeld, M. (1982). A model for activity intervention in disaster-stricken communities. *American Journal of Occupational Therapy*, *36*, 229-235.

Rosenfeld, M. (1984). Crisis intervention: the nuclear task approach. *American Journal of Occupational Therapy*, *38*, 382-385.

Rosenfeld, M. (in press). Occupational disruption and adaptation: a study of house fire victims. *American Journal of Occupational Therapy*.

Short, J. (1984). Changing role expectations of psychiatric occupational therapists. *Occupational Therapy in Mental Health*, *4*, pp. 19-27.

Tagore, R. (1928). *Fireflies*. New York: Macmillan.

The Promise of Occupational Therapy: Professional Challenges, Personal Rewards

Susan B. Fine, MA, OTR, FAOTA

SUMMARY. Personal reflections regarding the author's thirty year commitment to mental health practice are shared with a new generation of practitioners. The rapidly changing health care system, the versatility and richness of the specialty, and the availability of role models and mentors provide many promising opportunities for personal growth and professional satisfaction for those who choose to rise to the challenge.

INTRODUCTION

This article is an integration of two presentations. The first was to participants in the Fieldwork II Student Seminar on Mental Health Practice at The Payne Whitney Psychiatric Clinic during the summer of 1988. Its purpose: to highlight the integrative potential of this specialty for professional and personal development. The second was as Mentor for The Susan B. Fine Class of 1989, University of Texas Medical Branch at Galveston on November 12, 1988. On this occasion the author had the special honor and complex task of capturing elements of the "mentoring" process in a single two hour presentation. The remarks that follow reflect a reconstruction drawn from both efforts. While liberties have been taken with the original material in the interest of cohesion and readability, the first and

Susan B. Fine, recipient of the Eleanor Clark Slagle Lectureship for 1990, is director of therapeutic activities at the Payne Whitney Psychiatric Clinic, New York Hospital-Cornell Medical Center and senior lecturer in psychiatry, Cornell Medical College.

second person format has been preserved to emphasize the personal nature of this intergenerational exchange.

THE TASK: YOUR FUTURE/MY PAST

Addressing a new generation of practitioners is both a pleasure and a challenge. In welcoming you to the profession I have the luxury of directing your attention to issues and values that hold meaning for me. Hopefully, there is adequate synchrony between the needs and interests of reader and author. That is, after all, the principle purpose of intergenerational presentations such as these, to establish a connection, to suggest a path, to offer a "model," perhaps even to inspire as others have inspired us.

There is a belief that age and experience bring with them wisdom, insight and skill. Those who recognize the limitations and exceptions to this homily are perhaps the most wise and insightful. Nonetheless, tradition, scholars, and our own experience indicate that role models and mentors can play a very special part in our professional "coming of age." Role models provide us with an example of standards, skills and qualities we wish to acquire. A mentor, in a more active and conscious mode, serves as teacher-sponsor-host-guide-exemplar and counselor (Rogers, 1986), someone who imparts experience and knowledge, and helps to acculturate you into your new role over time. Under the usual circumstances of mentoring, each of you would play a more active role in selecting an individual whose experience and style might enrich your professional development. Someone whose vision of, and action in the field strikes a meaningful chord. Someone who is willing and able to engage in this complex nurturing, information-giving and advisory relationship. Although I obviously cannot provide you with the longer term collaboration that mentoring implies, perhaps we can touch upon some useful elements of the process.

What *can* I offer you in such a brief contact? Thirty years of experience? That could be very boring. However, some thoughts about what has made OT engaging enough to *sustain* thirty years of commitment might be worth sharing. Therefore, what follows are some personal reflections about professional themes and issues that I believe to be critical elements of our work, of our professional mission, and our professional self-esteem. They have strongly influenced my career and view of occupational therapy. Perhaps they will be useful for you as well.

A basic theme in occupational therapy is "integration," as in: "making whole, bringing all the parts together; the organization of organic, psychological or social traits and tendencies into a harmonious whole (Webster, 1984)." This concept should be most familiar through the bio-psycho-social treatment model. However, I wish to broaden its application beyond our work with patients to two other spheres: our roles and relationships within the health care system; and our personal roles, skills and growth over the course of our careers. The theme of integration can serve as a useful motif for recognizing the versatility and richness of occupational therapy, for understanding the importance of establishing a more central, influential role for yourselves in the health care system, and for consciously charting the path of a dynamic, changing and fulfilling professional life.

When I entered Columbia University's School of Occupational Therapy in 1957, with a BA degree in fine arts and psychology from Brooklyn College, I was in search of some vehicle for integrating interests in the creative process and the way in which art reflected "matters of the mind," as they were understood during that psychoanalytic era. An interest in art therapy and a fortuitous opportunity to do volunteer work with an accommodating occupational therapist in a geriatric center during my senior college year, in fact, were what brought me to OT. This contact with disoriented, but responsive residents and a supportive supervising therapist was moving, enlightening, and timely. It anchored my enthusiasm for analytic insight and the power of the unconscious with reality and heretofore illusive information about what occupational therapy was. It broadened my narrow and naive view of the potential of activity as therapy and taught me that the patient was more than his illness.

At Columbia, a fascination with the medical milieu and a surprising facility with "the sciences" fueled recurring fantasies of attending medical school. However, matters of the mind and a stronger sense of myself as a "helper" than a "scientist" won out. A two hour lecture on psychiatric OT by an inspiring professional greatly influenced that decision. That was to be the first of many contacts with Gail Fidler, the role model and mentor who influenced my early professional development and longer term commitment to the field. Needless to say our relationship extended beyond those two hours. Even after 30 years, and numerous collaborations, I continue to feel indebted to her for the skillful guiding, nurturing and role modeling that launched my career.

What was so special about Gail? Besides being smart, articulate and feisty, she had a *conviction* about OT and she was not afraid to share it. She had a *vision* of OT and she found pleasure in *thinking* it through and testing out *both* the science and the art. She saw the effort required to convey her beliefs as *challenges worth pursuing* . . . lonely as it sometimes was. While she certainly provided me with a preliminary "map" of the terrain of mental health practice and an exceptional "model" for professional thought and action, the most potent message she conveyed to me was *the promise of OT* and *the promise of me*: what I could perhaps become.

Promise, in this context, brings with it no assurances, as in the making of a promise. It is intended to reflect the *potential* of our field; its impact on our patients; its impact on the health care system; and its impact on *you*, as individuals whose commitment, longevity and output will be heavily influenced by the field's capacity to fill your changing needs. Therein lies the meaning of this paper's title, The Promise of OT: Professional Challenges, Personal Rewards.

THE CHALLENGES

Challenges come in all sizes and shapes. The very nature of our mission, to facilitate independent function, is a challenge. So is the complicated difficult patient, the complicated difficult physician, and the complicated difficult supervisor. However, the greatest challenge facing you as you embark upon your career is the changing face of the health care system. The system is the stage on which you will practice. It establishes powerful ground rules; it can be a source of support and status; and, it can also be a source of great deal of anxiety.

It seems fitting to describe the health care system with an illness metaphor. It has multiple lesions, it is acutely symptomatic, and it is undergoing radical surgery. Reimbursement is being curtailed, lengths of stay are getting shorter and shorter, services are being reduced, and training programs are at risk. While the major symptom (unbearably high costs) has been targeted for excision, the complex underlying causes and effects of cost cutting are not receiving enough attention. It's only fair to ask: Will "this patient" survive? How skilled and objective are those performing the procedure? What residual effects or disabilities will there be? What will health care look like and how effectively will it resume its role and fulfill its mission after discharge?

Belabored as this metaphor may be, it serves to highlight the nature of our profession's concerns and the many challenges that await you. Where will we be during and after this extended health care crisis? The powerful economic, scientific and social trends of today and tomorrow are dynamic and changing forces that influence the focus, quantity and quality of our relationships with patients and colleagues. They effect our status and professional sense of self as we respond to increasing competition from a great array of professional and paraprofessional groups, to demands for research and outcome data, and to pressures to expand our skills beyond "helper" to a more versatile clinician-scientist-entrepreneur-politician (Fine, 1988).

There are those who might tell you your timing's off; you've picked a chaotic period in which to enter a health and human services field. They may be right. There are others who will warn you of the turbulence, teach you the fundamental clinical skills of your profession, and send you off to do your thing. There is certainly nothing wrong with entering the marketplace with the basic tools of your trade. There is, however, a third perspective that says there's *more* to practice today than fundamental clinical skills. Any vision you may have of a seemingly simple, unidimensional relationship with a client in need, with muscles or egos to be strengthened, is *too* narrow a vision. That patient sets in motion a complex range of questions that will move you into areas far beyond muscles and egos. You need to be prepared. You need to see yourself as increasingly competent to answer such questions as: What is the patient getting for his money? How much of it does he really need now?

What impact will it have on him? How long will it take? What is the least restrictive and least costly environment in which to provide these services? Who provides the service best (Fine, 1986)?

The ghosts of many elements of the system will accompany you into your treatment clinic. There will be other members of the team, the often reductionistic biomedical model, hospital administrators, third party payers and accreditation surveyors, all with missions and varying degrees of power . . . brokering for the shrinking piece of the financial pie. They are our "partners" in the rehabilitation process, although not always sympathetic or supportive of our perspective and our priorities. Patients will not always be cooperative or grateful for your efforts either. Your concept of purposeful activity may not be theirs. They want an outcome that makes a difference in their lives. You must be prepared to work with them in clarifying what that is, translating it into realistic and reasonable goals, and pursuing it with knowledge, skill and speed. While all of this is going on, new knowledge will constantly emerge and reshape the form and substance of what you believed to be the state of the art.

Occupational therapy's emergence from the nineties as a major force in rehabilitation, prevention and health maintenance, will be greatly determined by *your* capacities to rise to these many challenges. This requires more than good clinical instincts and a belief in the potential of purposeful activity. It is more complex than assessing negative symptoms of schizophrenia or developing a prevocational program. It certainly transcends the area of specialization you will soon be selecting. And, in doing so, it provides you with superb opportunities for personal and professional development that can take you far beyond your current expectations.

CHALLENGES AS STIMULANTS FOR CHANGE AND GROWTH

While todays challenges are big time challenges, they have without a doubt pushed us (as individual practitioners and as an organized profession) to anticipate, think, plan and act far more forcefully and effectively than we might otherwise have done. We have learned, as you will learn, that challenges can serve as powerful stimulants for managing change in the system, in occupational therapy practice, and in yourselves. "Manage" does not mean "getting by." It means adopting a problem-solving perspective that can harness the more productive potentials of this period. It is, what I've referred to elsewhere as, "working the system" (Fine, 1988).

This means making the most of trends by monitoring and understanding them, assuming a proactive stance, and *using* them to advantage by spotlighting our assets and creating a market wherever possible. An excellent example of "working the system" is the 1988 symposium on Access to Quality Care in Rehabilitation, organized by The American Occupational Therapy Association and cosponsored by eleven other organizations. This potentially powerful coalition of specialists were brought together by our national leadership to examine factors preventing access to rehabilitation services. By first identifying and exploring key policy issues impeding access, they have begun the formidable but important task of problem-solving through a new and larger constituency and network of resources than we could have generated on our own. The Association has drawn attention to occupational therapy, showcased its leadership capacities and knowledge, while developing a marketing strategy for rehabilitation. This coalition will be in a useful position to lobby on the Hill, negotiate with the government for health care scholarships and with the insurance industry for increased reimbursement.

Another example of making the most of trends is the identification and marketing of "brief focused rehabilitation" as a relevant occupational therapy strategy for patients during short term, acute care psychiatric hospitalizations. Unenlightened views of psychiatric rehabilitation and beliefs that medication and crisis intervention alone adequately prepare patients for rapid community re-entry have limited access to needed services in many acute care settings. The rationale for brief focused rehabilitation, the "time limited, task and goal directed learning of self-management skills" (Fine, in press) provides a systematic reasoning process for the delivery of realistic, necessary services that enhance adaptive capacities, prepare patients for discharge and tenure in the community, and may well reduce the likelihood of costly rehospitalizations. The marketing of brief focused rehabilitation in interdisciplinary conferences and journals gives visibility to the value of occupational therapy by translating its focus, methods and objectives into language that is compatible with the aspirations of consumers, the cost concerns of third party payers, and the goals and realities of acute care settings. Careful documentation and objective data collection are, of course, the ultimate test of value. Such endeavors are under way in a variety of settings, but must be undertaken by more therapists, in more clinical centers, more rapidly.

RISING TO THE CHALLENGE

The inclination to rise to the personal and professional challenges before us involves a view of life to which we are not all born. There are those of us who see the glass half empty while others view it as half full. Moreover, not all of us have identified "systems management" as an expected element of our daily working life. Those muscles and egos seem formidable enough, certainly at this juncture in your professional lives.

The phenomena of viewing change as challenge is an element of personality that has been studied and called "hardiness" (Kobasa, 1979). Researchers examining the relationship of hardiness to stress induced illness, conclude that this adaptive style, defined by such personality variables as commitment, control and challenge, protect the individual from illness. I believe it also protects one from professional burn-out. Our conscious efforts to understand and cultivate hardiness in ourselves, as we negotiate the system, is as important as our efforts to cultivate it in our patients. Who is it that responds to the challenge of damaged muscles and walks again? Who overcomes recurring episodes of depression and rebuilds a manageable and meaningful life? Who rises to the threat of constraining reimbursement regulations by clarifying occupational therapy as an active and reimbursable treatment agent?

For those who are "hardy," *commitment* is expressed as a tendency to involve oneself in, rather than experience alienation from, whatever one is doing. They have a generalized sense of purpose that allows them to find events, things and people in their environment meaningful. They are sufficiently invested in themselves and their work, family and friends to not easily give up under pressure.

They are active and approach situations rather than respond with avoidance or passivity.

The *control* element of hardiness is expressed by feeling and acting as if one is influential, rather than helpless, in the face of problems. This involves the perception of oneself as having influence through the use of imagination, knowledge, skill and choice.

The *challenge* variable is expressed as a belief that change, rather than stability, is normal in life and that the anticipation of changes are interesting incentives for growth rather than threats to security.

Although the sources of hardiness are not fully understood, personality theories dealing with competency suggest that strong tendencies toward commitment, control and challenge have their origins in early experiences with a variety and diversity of events, from stimulation and support for exercising symbolization, imagination and judgment, from approval and admiration for doing things oneself, and from role models who advocate hardiness and show it in their own functioning (Kobasa, 1978).

This formulation is of special significance in our relationships with patients. The rehabilitation process is characterized by an optimism and persistence reflected in the belief that assets and liabilities can be harnessed and mobilized in the interest of adaptation. We presume our patients can, within reason, move beyond their illness and disability to maximize independent functioning. We pursue that mission by helping them to acquire or reactivate the requisite attitudes and skills. Shouldn't we expect ourselves to apply that same tenacity in other relationships in the system? Shouldn't we cultivate elements of hardiness as an essential basic professional skill? Wasn't an aspect of what I saw and admired in Gail Fidler hardiness? Surely her love of challenge and change, her many scholarly efforts to define and develop practice and promote recognition for the field reflect that. Moreover, her ability to nurture and support those independent behaviors in others has contributed to a large cohort of hardy, tenacious professionals who have found rewards while rising to the challenges.

When I returned to full time hospital based practice after nine years in part-time ventures as educator, consultant, graduate student and private practitioner while starting my family, I struggled with my reluctance to become more manager than clinician. As I became "the boss" in a new era characterized by: thirty day rather than two year lengths of stay, a focus on function rather than the unconscious, and the growth of multidisciplinary activity therapy programs rather than occupational therapy departments, I soon realized that the changes and challenges before me were responsive to the same energetic problem-solving process I valued so highly in clinical tasks. It was as relevant and as rewarding in program and staff development, supervision, interdisciplinary struggles, and systems management. I was not giving up skills, knowledge and satisfaction, but rather expanding and integrating them in another context, at a different level, and assuredly, at a different pace.

REWARDS

What about the rewards? They also come in all sizes and shapes. They are best appraised by the individual, since each of us want and need different things at different points in our lives. Just as we look for the "fit" between our patient's needs and the treatment task, so we must expect to identify the fit between our changing needs and the field's and system's opportunities. These are some you might want to try on for size:

- Rewards come from finishing your final requirements for graduation and licensure.
- Rewards come from the resistant patient who one day says, "I was just wishing you'd come."
- Rewards come when you've struggled to speak up at a time meeting and the preoccupied resident listens long enough to tell you that your functional assessment is what got the patient into the right residential treatment program before the insurance ran out.
- Rewards come from being looked up to by *your* first fieldwork student.
- Rewards come from colleagues' recognition after your first conference presentation.
- Rewards come from the pleasure and surprise of receiving a research grant.
- Rewards come from discovering that leadership capacities are

not limited to those in leadership positions, and that you have some.

- Rewards come when your family *finally* understands what occupational therapy is.
- Rewards come from discovering that your professional organizations and a virtual army of volunteers are out there advocating and establishing credibility for what you do.
- Rewards come from joining them and demonstrating that you too can "work the system."
- Rewards come from knowing that we have a strong and lengthy commitment to rehabilitation at a time when functional performance and skills of daily living are identified as outcomes of major interest to consumers.
- Rewards come from the extraordinary professional opportunities that far exceed our numbers and are waiting to be seized.
- Rewards, as you can see, come from *getting* as well as giving. While this may sound antagonistic to the instincts that drew you to this helping profession, "getting" is an important element of professionalism and personal satisfaction. As a predominantly female profession imbedded in traditions that are still a product of a pre-liberation era, we continue to be heavily influenced by notions of power, acceptance and success as acquired through giving and interdependence. Be assured that professional achievement at all levels requires *getting as well as giving*, and *independent as well as interdependent* modes of behavior (Fine 1987).
- Rewards emerge from the very same diversity that can sometimes be distorted into our "being all things to all people." However, the field's diversity has served me well for 30 years, allowing me to have a career in a career in a career: clinician, teacher, administrator, author, researcher and mentor. Diversity has fostered the integration of seemingly disparate aspects of myself, harnessing intellectual and academic inclinations through writing and research, without diminishing a very strong commitment to the interpersonal and the nurturing of change in others. While I am still a "helper" in my clinical, supervisory and collegial relationships, I have also found the right opportunities to cultivate the science and art of occupa-

tional therapy. While "doing battle" with the medical model in the conference rooms of my clinic and national interdisciplinary forums when necessary, I am also advocating for a realistic and effective partnership between medical and rehabilitation approaches, recognizing full well that the success of these interventions rests in our abilities to overcome "turf" and meet the patients' bio-psychosocial needs.

THE ULTIMATE TEST

I often joke about what I'll be "when I grow up." Although the world and its opportunities have changed significantly since 1959, I believe I would, once again, choose psychiatric occupational therapy. If I were to identify the singularly most remarkable element characterizing my tenure in this specialty, it would be that I've never been bored . . . at least not for long. There have always been purposeful, professional activities to pursue and master. There have always been challenges and changes that test and expand my knowledge, skill, sense of mastery and choice. There have always been extraordinary people, patients and professionals, whose courage, integrity and commitment to "rising above adversity" continue to be an inspiration.

As you move out into the real world of occupational therapy practice, no doubt hoping for a bit more stability than change, I wish you well. May you find as much personal satisfaction as I have; may you discover the promise in OT . . . and the hardiness in yourselves.

REFERENCES

Fine, S.B. (1986) Trends in mental health. In SCOPE Curriculum Manual, S. Robertson (Ed.), Rockville MD: The American Occupational Therapy Association. 19-32.
Fine, S.B. (1987) Looking ahead: Opportunities for occupational therapy in the next decade. Occupational Therapy in Mental Health, Vol 7(4), Winter, 3-12.
Fine, S.B. (1988) Nationally Speaking Column. Working the system: A perspective for managing change. American Journal of Occupational Therapy. Vol 42(7), July, 417-426.

Fine, S.B. (In press) Brief focused rehabilitation: Strategies for short-term psychiatric settings.

Kobasa, S.C. (1979) Stressful life events, personality, and health: An inquiry into hardiness. Journal of Personality and Social Psychology. Vol 37(1), January, 1-11.

Rogers, J.C. (1986) Nationally Speaking: Mentoring for career achievement and advancement. American Journal of Occupational Therapy. Vol 40(2), February, 79-82.

Webster's II (1984) New Riverside University Dictionary. Boston: Houghton Mifflin Co.

Reflections on Choice

Gail S. Fidler, OTR, FAOTA

SUMMARY. The choices made throughout one's career clearly shape the destiny of that career and impact the profession. The breadth of options and one's choices are markedly influenced by one's value system and concomitant expectations. Certain beliefs and attitudes are especially relevant to and significant for women and thus a predominantly women's profession. Examination of some of these variables of choice, it is suggested, will expand vision and enable more productive and intrinsically gratifying choices.

The dictionary identifies the synonyms for choice as including: option, discrimination, determination, preference, volition, decision, judgment and dilemma. On reflection, each of us is able to associate with the experience characterized in these terms. Frequently we experience making a choice as a dilemma. Just as frequently perhaps, we take action or not, unaware that an option exists or that a choice has actually been made.

I am reminded of a story about a Catholic priest and a fundamentalist preacher who were seated side by side on an airplane. When they were asked about beverage choice, the priest ordered scotch and water and invited the preacher to join him. The preacher looked with horror at the priest exclaiming, "Father, I would rather commit adultery than have alcohol pass my lips." To which the priest replied, "Hmmm – did not realize I had such a choice!"

The other dimension of choice is, of course, the old adage that to not decide is to decide. There are always many more alternatives available to us than we are aware of or able at times to acknowledge. For a variety of social, cultural and personal reasons, we

Gail S. Fidler is Private Practicing Consultant, Mental Health and Rehabilitation, 362 Old York Road, Flemington, NJ 08822.

learn to limit our vision of possibilities. Additionally, our assessment of the alternatives we do see and the choices we make are equally influenced by the same social, cultural and personal values and beliefs. We know that increasing our awareness of options increases opportunity. That increased freedom to assess available alternatives and to act, enhances the possibility of opportunities being realized. Perhaps confronting and clarifying some of our traditional expectations, values and beliefs will help to move us toward this end.

For members of an evolving and predominantly women's profession, certain beliefs and values take on special significance in terms of choice and the impact of such choice on the practitioner and on the profession. What then are some of these attitudes and values which I believe are of particular importance to us.

First, and perhaps most fundamental is how we view RESPONSIBILITY FOR SELF. Each of us is more responsible than not for the events and quality of our life. We are not passive recipients but rather active agents in shaping our destiny. It is not so much what happens to us as it is what, by choice, we cause to happen. It is what we do about circumstances, about the other, the event, the system, that shapes our life.

This orientation, I suggest, is an inherent part of our values regarding personal freedom, freedom to choose our own way. As Carl Rodgers (1969) has stated:

> It is the realization that I can live myself, here and now, by my own choice — It is the burden of being responsible for the self one chooses to be — the recognition of a person that he is an emerging process, not a static end product — It is the quality of courage which enables a person to step into the uncertainty of the unknown.

The alternatives we see, the decisions we make are certainly shaped by where each of us stands in regard to such a value.

Closely related in many ways is the question of AUTONOMY. This involves one's personal orientation to self determination and one's need to feel in control of the events of one's life. In recent years the meaning and significance of autonomy has occupied an important place in research. Goleman (1986) has reported that research is demonstrating that the need to feel in control is universal and a critical factor in one's state of mental and physical health. Of special significance in this research is the evidence of a difference among people in the intensity of need, the relationship of the level of need to job and life style choice, satisfaction and sense of competence.

Coming to understand the degree of one's own need to be in control, addressing the values we hold regarding self determination and our right to value and exercise autonomy, are important variables of productive choice. When our beliefs and expectations limit our options, our sense of autonomy is threatened. I have, for example, regularly advised students and staff that by and large "an employer should always need you more than you need that employment." When the situation is perceived as reversed, one's options begin to be limited. Choices begin to focus on security and accommodation, the feeling of being "locked-in" grows and one's sense of autonomy is threatened or lost. How would our choices, our actions look if we acted on our need to be in control?

Let us look now at the belief, the expectation that anything one chooses to do for any length of time, especially one's work should be more fun, more INTRINSICALLY GRATIFYING than not. That perspective would certainly alter some of our decisions, would it not?

Again Goleman (1986) has reported that research regarding life satisfaction has cast doubts on our long held beliefs about those factors which determine satisfaction. Rather than approaching one's ego ideal or achieving one's life goal or dream, current research has identified quite different factors. The most critical factor, according to this report is the time spent in doing things which the individual finds meaningful, is most competent at and takes the most pleasure in. The critical elements for identifying what is most meaningful are described as (1) avoiding roles in life in which one experiences undesirable feelings, especially dependency and selfishness (not contributing to others) and (2) maintaining a distance from those things, those feeling states and activities that one abhors!

Such findings support the value of intrinsic gratification and enjoyment, do they not? We seem to hold to the ethic that pursuit of personal satisfaction is a selfish, self-serving motive unless it is related to giving to others. Many years ago I was privileged to learn from the eminent Dr. Harry Stack Sullivan. He consistently reinforced the concept that one cannot give what one does not have: that in essence, if you do not love or respect yourself, you do not have love or respect to give. Thus, selfishness, the lack of regard for others is a lack of regard for self.

Our attitudes and beliefs concerning FAILURE have a decided influence on the options we are able to consider. A fear of failure limits options, makes risk taking frightening and generates passivity. Bennis and Nanus (1985) quote J. H. Johnson, the publisher of *Ebony* as saying, "Most people don't really believe in success. They feel helpless before they start—we have the power to make it—it's the fear of failure that gets in the way."

These same authors report that the most impressive quality of the 90 top leaders they studied was the way they responded to failure. Most never thought about it or when they did, it was in the context of a normal set of expectations. An acceptance of the reality that some times you win, some times you don't. These successful leaders talked about a "glitch," a set back, false start, error, mess, but never failures. It was simply not part of their vocabulary.

Is it not puzzling, considering how much we learn from our errors or "glitches," how they are so frequently the beginning of new learning, a new start or discovery, that we continue to consider such happenings failure? What values and beliefs continue to warn us about risk, about failure and thus influence our choices?

Bennis and Nanus (1985) suggest that fear of failure relates to two perspectives. They identify these are one's self regard and one's expectations about the outcome of the event. The self regard issue is of course the question of how competent we believe we are. These authors say that when a person doesn't try or gives up an option because they doubt they can do what is required, such decisions reflect a negative self regard. On the other hand they state that when a person doesn't try or gives up because they expect that their effort will not change things, or when they alter their decisions because of a fear of criticism or retaliation, these are inhibitions resulting from expectations about outcomes. Beck and Hillman (1986), Peters and Waterman (1982) and Kantor (1984) all provide ample evidence of the relationship of these factors to choice, decision making and achievement.

CONFRONTATION, what this means to us, what expectations we have about outcomes from such encounters, certainly influences our preference of one choice over another. Do our values tell us that confrontation is a negative act which will almost inevitably result in angry retaliation? Have we learned to fear and avoid it? Or have we come to view confrontation as positive behavior which clarifies relationships and expectations between ourselves and others? When seen from this latter perspective, confrontation reflects a set of beliefs about the legitimacy of the interests and perceptions of others and one's self. It conveys the expectation that change is valued and always possible and that open, direct communication demonstrates a respect for and a caring about the integrity of self and other. When we do not confront a person or a situation, we most likely are giving a message that says, "I don't really care" or "It's not important."

Beck and Hillmar (1986) believe that confrontation when viewed as positive, reflects a number of values which are expressed as: I accept your wants and interests as legitimate and speak up for mine; I care enough about you to give you an opportunity to change once you are aware of the problem or concern; I care enough about the success of this organization to confront any behavior that I view as damaging to it; and finally, I care about me and avoidance of confrontation causes me discomfort, anger and guilt which inhibit my effectiveness and my sense of satisfaction.

The traditional socialization process of most women ill prepares us to accept confrontation as a positive value.

It is unlikely that any one would speak of choices, decisions and values without addressing POWER. Power is the essence of getting things accomplished, of causing things to happen. How we experience power, how we understand our own, our comfort in using what power we have and how we view the difference between our power and that of others, shape how we assess alternatives and choose to act or not to act. Harragan (1977) and Henning and Jardin

(1977) provide challenging evidence of how many of our values as women develop and the influence of these values on our behavior and expectations.

Power is viewed by some of us as forcefulness and synonymous with authority, position, control over another, law and enforcement. Others have come to value power as positive ways of influencing others, as effective energy and capability. Bennis and Nanus (1985) believe power is the empowerment of self and others so as to translate intention into reality.

Beck and Hillmar (1986) point out that the empowerment of self is an incremental process of learning how to use one's personal and professional resources more fully. They identify the elements of this process as including the pursuit of self growth, increasing one's competence, using and developing the power that one has, becoming more aware of what is happening, knowing what one wants and asking for it, speaking out to identify one's own position and finally practicing positive confrontation.

The capacity to empower others relates to our values and expectations about others but most particularly to how we view ourselves, to our values of self. Rodgers (1961) expressed this theme by saying, "the degree to which we can create relationships which facilitate the growth of others, is in measure to the growth in self which we have achieved." Bennis and Nanus (1985) emphasize this belief by recounting a delightful ancient Chinese story.

> When Yen Ho was about to take up his duties as tutor to the heir of Ling — he went to an old wise man for advice. 'I have to deal, he said, with a man of depraved and murderous disposition — How is one to deal with a man of this sort?' 'I'm glad you asked replied the sage — The first thing you must do is not to improve him — but to improve yourself!

A positive SELF REGARD is a critical force in expanding our options and enabling productive choices. It is evident that the values and attitudes which I have briefly addressed are indeed interrelated with our self concept. A positive regard for self develops out of the pursuit of self growth, a search for knowledge and understanding about self. This ongoing process involves: clarifying our values; testing the efficacy of our expectations; increasing our awareness of our feelings, thoughts and actions; clarifying our relationships with others; identifying and perfecting our competencies, and identifying and managing our limitations.

Every so often we need to be reminded that a positive self regard emerges from verification of our strengths and competencies, not from evidence of our inadequacies. I have come to believe that a healthy, objective recognition and management of individual limitations becomes possible only as we are able to acknowledge and affirm our competencies. We accept this concept and operationalize it with patients but we seem to have a somewhat different standard for ourselves and others.

The quest for understanding others, for developing an interpersonal intelligence and skill is a dimension of the quest for self growth and positive self regard. Interpersonal competence and a positive concept of self are inseparable. There is no such thing as a onesided coin!

Taking another and final page from Bennis and Nanus (1985), they relate that the top leaders whom they studied used five key interpersonal skills. They describe these skills as the ability to:

— accept people as they are, not as you would like them to be.
— enter the skin of the other.
— approach relationships in terms of the present rather than the past.
— treat those close to you with the same attention that you extend to strangers or acquaintances, not taking persons for granted.
— trust others. The risk of being deceived is wiser than taking for granted that others are insincere or incompetent.
— do without constant approval, especially at work.

The nature of learning about self and others in the process of developing such skills is quite clear. Equally clear is the impact that such learning and practice would have on expanding our options and increasing our potential for making productive choices. The expectations we have about our selves, about others and our external world, our values and attitudes, shape and influence the options we see and the decisions we make. The choices which you will continue to make in terms of your practice as an Occupational Therapist will unquestionably shape the fabric of your career and of your profession.

REFERENCES

Beck, A.C., & Hillmar, E.D. (1986). Positive management Practices. San Francisco: Jossey-Bass.

Bennis, W., Nanus, B. (1985). Leaders: The strategies for charge. New York: Harper & Row.

Harragan, B.L. (1977). Games mother never taught you. New York: Warner Books.

Hennig, M., & Jardin, A. (1977). The managerial woman. New York: Anchor Press/Doubleday.

Kantor, R.M. (1984). The change masters. New York: Simon and Shuster.

Goleman, D. (1986, October 7). Feeling of control viewed as central in mental health. *The New York Times*, PP. C1,C11.

Goleman, D. (1986, December 23). Meaningful activities and temperament key in satisfaction with life. *The New York Times*, PP. C1,C8.

Peters, T.J., Waterman, R.H. (1982). In search of excellence. New York: Warner Books.

Rodgers, C. (1969). Freedom to learn. Columbus, Ohio: Charles E. Merrill, pp. 268-269.

Rodgers, C. (1961). On becoming a person. Boston: Houghton Mifflin.